W9-DGI-367

Richard Hoefer, PhD
James Midgley, PhD
Editors

International Perspectives on Welfare to Work Policy

International Perspectives on Welfare to Work Policy has been co-published simultaneously as *Journal of Policy Practice*, Volume 5, Numbers 2/3 2006.

Pre-publication
REVIEWS,
COMMENTARIES,
EVALUATIONS . . .

"TIMELY . . . The RESEARCH IS SOUND AND THE BOOK IS CLEARLY AND EFFECTIVELY WRITTEN for use by social welfare scholars."

Leon Ginsberg, PhD, former Dean
College of Social Work
University of South Carolina

"In the past two decades, there have been significant changes in the social welfare states of the developed world. Those at the bottom—unemployed youth, long-term unemployed, lone parents, immigrants, and other "socially excluded"–are no longer entitled to income support but now must engage in work or work-related activities, called "activation" or "workfare." The world has changed from "entitlements" to "responsibilities." This collection of essays dealing with the United States, the United Kingdom, and Hong Kong, raises the important question of the role of professional social work. In most instances, social workers have not played a central role in these changes or in welfare reform generally. The authors argue, using many excellent examples, that the social work profession has a great deal to contribute to these developments."

Joel F. Handler, JD
Richard C. Maxwell Professor of Law
School of Public Affairs
UCLA School of Law

"Provides a basic introduction to welfare-to-work policies and practices as viewed from the perspective of the social work profession. . . . Describes some of the major policy developments in the U.S. as well as selected measures created under the rubric of social activation and inclusion in the U.K., Australia, and Hong Kong. These comparative examples create an opportunity for readers to explore specific facets of welfare-to-work policy in different national contexts. Authors in this volume raise questions about the relevance of social work in advancing, implementing, and alternatively, opposing welfare-to-work in its various forms. They consider whether and how social workers should engage in workfare policies and practice. Some authors issue an explicit challenge to the social work profession to attend to this significant feature of the contemporary welfare state."

Evelyn Z. Brodkin, PhD
Political Science, MIT,
Associate Professor,
University of Chicago, School of Social Service Administration

The Haworth Press, Inc.

International Perspectives on Welfare to Work Policy

International Perspectives on Welfare to Work Policy has been co-published simultaneously as *Journal of Policy Practice,* Volume 5, Numbers 2/3 2006.

Monographic Separates from *Journal of Policy Practice*™

For additional information on these and other Haworth Press titles, including descriptions, tables of contents, reviews, and prices, use the QuickSearch catalog at http://www.HaworthPress.com.

Journal of Policy Practice is the successor title to *The Social Policy Journal*,* which changed title after Volume 4, No. 3/4, 2005. *Journal of Policy Practice*, under its new title, began with Volume 5, No.1, 2006.

International Perspectives on Welfare to Work Policy, edited by Richard Hoefer, PhD, and James Midgley, PhD (Vol. 5, No. 2/3, 2006). *"Timely . . . The research is sound and the book is clearly and effectively written for use by social welfare scholars." (Leon Ginsberg, PhD, former Dean, College of Social Work, University of South Carolina)*

Cutting-Edge Social Policy Research, *edited by Richard Hoefer, PhD (Vol. 4, No. 3/4, 2005). "A valuable read for social work scholars and practitioners. Richard Hoefer's craft as an editor is clear in the choice that he makes to include a broad range of contributions that address the needs of at-risk populations, from children who are abused, to adults seeking to maintain their quality of life. He wisely selects multiple research designs that represent best practices in scientific inquiry, including program evaluation, qualitative, and quantitative methodologies." (Deborah Stutevant, PhD, Professor of Theology and Social Work, Hope College)*

International Perspectives
on Welfare to Work Policy

Richard Hoefer, PhD
James Midgley, PhD
Editors

International Perspectives on Welfare to Work Policy has been
co-published simultaneously as *Journal of Policy Practice,*
Volume 5, Numbers 2/3 2006.

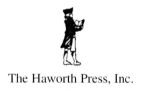

The Haworth Press, Inc.

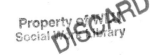

New York • London • Victoria (AU)
www.HaworthPress.com

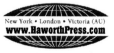

International Perspectives on Welfare to Work Policy has been co-published simultaneously as *Journal of Policy Practice*™, Volume 5, Numbers 2/3 2006.

Cover design by Kerry Mack

Library of Congress Cataloging-in-Publication Data

International perspectives on welfare to work policy / Richard Hoefer, James Midgley, Editors.
    p. cm.
    Includes bibliographical references and index.
    Co-published simultaneously as Journal of policy practice, volume 5, numbers 2/3 2006.
    ISBN-13: 978-0-7890-3367-3 (hard cover : alk. paper)
    ISBN-10: 0-7890-3367-4 (hard cover : alk. paper)
    ISBN-13: 978-0-7890-3368-0 (soft cover : alk. paper)
    ISBN-10: 0-7890-3368-2 (soft cover : alk. paper)
    1. Welfare recipients–Employment–Cross-cultural studies. 2. Public welfare–Cross-cultural studies. 3. Social policy–Cross-cultural studies. I. Hoefer, Richard. II. Midgley, James. III. Journal of policy practice.
    HV69.I57 2006
    362.5'84–dc22
                                                         2006001668

Indexing, Abstracting & Website/Internet Coverage

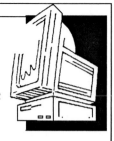

This section provides you with a list of major indexing & abstracting services and other tools for bibliographic access. That is to say, each service began covering this periodical during the year noted in the right column. Most Websites which are listed below have indicated that they will either post, disseminate, compile, archive, cite or alert their own Website users with research-based content from this work. (This list is as current as the copyright date of this publication.)

Abstracting, Website/Indexing Coverage . . . . Year When Coverage Began

- *CareData: the database supporting social care management and practice <http://www.elsc.org.uk/caredata/caredata.htm>* 2002

- *CINAHL (Cumulative Index to Nursing & Allied Health Literature), in print, EBSCO, and SilverPlatter, DataStar, and PaperChase. (Support materials include Subject Heading List, Database Search Guide, and instructional video) <http://www.cinahl.com>* 2003

- *Criminal Justice Abstracts* 2003

- *DH-Data (available via DataStar and in the HMIC [Health Management Information Consortium] (CD ROM)* 2003

- *Educational Administration Abstracts (EAA)* 2002

- *Elsevier Scopus <http://www.info.scopus.com>* 2005

- *e-psyche, LLC <http://www.e-psyche.net>* 2002

- *Family & Society Studies Worldwide <http://www.nisc.com>* . . . 2002

- *Family Index Database <http://www.familyscholar.com>* 2003

- *Family Violence & Sexual Assault Bulletin* 2002

- *Google <http://www.google.com>* 2004

(continued)

Special Bibliographic Notes related to special journal issues
(separates) and indexing/abstracting:

- indexing/abstracting services in this list will also cover material in any "separate" that is co-published simultaneously with Haworth's special thematic journal issue or DocuSerial. Indexing/abstracting usually covers material at the article/chapter level.
- monographic co-editions are intended for either non-subscribers or libraries which intend to purchase a second copy for their circulating collections.
- monographic co-editions are reported to all jobbers/wholesalers/approval plans. The source journal is listed as the "series" to assist the prevention of duplicate purchasing in the same manner utilized for books-in-series.
- to facilitate user/access services all indexing/abstracting services are encouraged to utilize the co-indexing entry note indicated at the bottom of the first page of each article/chapter/contribution.
- this is intended to assist a library user of any reference tool (whether print, electronic, online, or CD-ROM) to locate the monographic version if the library has purchased this version but not a subscription to the source journal.
- individual articles/chapters in any Haworth publication are also available through the Haworth Document Delivery Service (HDDS).

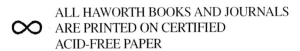

International Perspectives on Welfare to Work Policy

CONTENTS

ABOUT THE EDITORS

Richard Hoefer, PhD, is Associate Professor, School of Social Work, University of Texas at Arlington, Arlington, TX. He specializes in the areas of social policy and program administration, with a particular emphasis on advocacy and program evaluation. Dr. Hoefer was founding editor of *The Social Policy Journal*, and is editor of *Journal of Policy Practice*. He is the author of *Advocacy Practice for Social Justice* and numerous articles on topics such as advocacy, nonprofit management, and program evaluation.

James Midgley, PhD, is Harry and Riva Specht Professor of Public Social Services and Dean of the School of Social Welfare at the University of California, Berkeley. He has published widely on issues of social development and international social welfare. His most recent books include *Controversial Issues in Social Policy* (with Howard Karger and Brene Brown, Allyn & Bacon, 2003), *Social Policy for Development* (with Anthony Hall, Sage Publications, 2004) and *Lessons from Abroad: Adapting International Social Welfare Innovations* (with M. C. Hokenstad, NASW Press, 2004).

Introduction:
Social Workers
and Welfare to Work Programs:
International Perspectives

Richard Hoefer

James Midgley

As is well-known, social work emerged as an organized professional activity in Europe and North America in the late 19th century. Its founders were concerned with the social problems that accompanied industrialization and rapid urbanization at the time and believed that these could be addressed through professional intervention. Although some focused on specific social problems such as child abuse and neglect, mental illness, or family disintegration, the underlying problem was poverty and the first social workers inevitably dealt with families who were poor. They were also involved in the provision of poor relief in one form or another. In some cases, this involved the payment of small cash benefits while in others, material assistance in the form of food parcels, clothing and blankets was given.

Richard Hoefer is Associate Professor, School of Social Work, University of Texas at Arlington, Arlington, TX 76019 (E-mail: rhoefer@uta.edu). James Midgley is Dean and Specht Professor, School of Social Welfare, University of California, Berkeley, 120 Haviland Hall, Berkeley, CA 94704 (E-mail: swdean@berkeley.edu).

The authors are Editors of this volume.

[Haworth co-indexing entry note]: "Introduction: Social Workers and Welfare to Work Programs: International Perspectives." Hoefer, Richard, and James Midgley. Co-published simultaneously in *Journal of Policy Practice* (The Haworth Press, Inc.) Vol. 5, No. 2/3, 2006, pp. 1-6; and: *International Perspectives on Welfare to Work Policy* (ed: Richard Hoefer, and James Midgley) The Haworth Press, Inc., 2006, pp. 1-6. Single or multiple copies of this article are available for a fee from The Haworth Document Delivery Service [1-800-HAWORTH, 9:00 a.m. - 5:00 p.m. (EST). E-mail address: docdelivery@ haworthpress.com].

Available online at http://www.haworthpress.com/web/JPP
doi:10.1300/J508v05n02_01

1

However, as the founders of social work began to formalize their activities and to campaign for professionalization, they generally disavowed this type of poor relief and instead argued for the provision of advice and counseling which would help poor families to address their problems and become economically self-sufficient. This was the philosophy of the Charity Organization Society which laid great stress on interventions that would meet the underlying psychological and social needs of poor families. The organization's friendly visitors, as the first social workers were known, were required to make a diagnosis of the family's problems and formulate a treatment plan that would foster independent functioning. The organization was very critical of charities that provided "indiscriminate" material benefits to the poor, contending that this did little to address the underlying problems that were responsible for poverty.

Although the Charity Organization Society played a major role in shaping the emerging social work profession, other groups also contributed. For example, the settlement houses were also concerned with the problem of poverty but they did so at the neighborhood level stressing the need for interventions that organized local communities, offered sports and recreational activities, engaged in neighborhood improvement and provided adult education and other opportunities for poor people to improve their situation. They also believed that the middle-class university students who came to live and work in settlement houses would serve as role models and help those living in the slums realize their potential to improve themselves and secure a better quality of life. Like the caseworkers of the Charity Organization Society, settlement workers were not primarily concerned with material poor relief.

However, some of the early proponents of social work were in favor of interventions that dealt directly with material deprivation through the payment of income benefits. They urged the expansion and payment of more generous Poor Law benefits particularly to widows with children. The campaigns that resulted in the Mother's Pensions which were introduced by many state governments in the United States in the early 20th century are an example of this approach. Others argued for the abolition of means-tested benefits and the introduction of social insurance as well as demogrant child allowances that would subsidize the incomes of poor families. They also urged the expansion of public education, free health care and public housing all of which, they believed, would raise the incomes of poor families and create a more equal and fair society.

These different perspectives on how to deal with the poverty problem divided the founders of social work and there were sharp disagreements on the question of government intervention. Generally, the leaders of the Charity Organization Society and proponents of the emerging casework approach were opposed to statutory provisions directed at the poor. Although they did not reject the need for social reform, government programs, they believed, would foster dependency and have wider negative consequences for society as a whole. The leaders of the settlement movement were generally in favor of social reform but they continued to stress the need for community-based programs that mobilized local people and helped improve local social conditions. However, during the 20th century, government social programs did expand and, throughout the industrial world, statism eventually pervaded social welfare programs directed at the poor.

Despite the expansion of the statutory social services, the social work profession has maintained an ambivalent attitude towards statutory income support. The increasing specialization of social work and its articulation of distinctive fields of practice such as child welfare, disability, gerontology, mental health and medical social work, moved social caseworkers increasingly away from a concern with poverty. This trend was reinforced by the profession's adoption of psychoanalysis and other popular psychotherapies. As a result of these developments, many social workers failed to recognize that most of their clients were poor. They also failed to recognize that the specialized problems caseworkers were dealing with were, in fact, closely linked to an underlying condition of material deprivation.

However, it should be stressed that social work did not, as is often suggested, totally abandon the poor or forsake its original mission to serve the poor. Some social workers were directly involved in the creation of statutory income support programs and many supported the expansion of government social programs. In addition, some social workers found employment in government social service agencies responsible for the provision of income benefits. In some countries, social workers played a key role in managing these programs and linking them to other statutory social service programs that dealt with poor families.

But it cannot be claimed that the organized profession enthusiastically endorsed social work's involvement in statutory income support programs or regarded these services as a desirable arena for social work practice. Indeed, the public social services were often relegated in the profession's status hierarchy. Instead, social work practice in specialized nonprofit agencies, clinics and hospitals was regarded as more appropriate and, eventually, private psychotherapeutic practice emerged as the most prestigious, elite form of social work intervention.

Because relatively few social workers sought employment in statutory income support programs, these programs were not routinely administered by professional social workers even though the term social worker was widely used to describe those who undertook these tasks. Professionally qualified social workers may have occupied senior administrative and policy positions within government agencies responsible for these programs but, generally, the link between social work and income support and maintenance programs was tenuous. In addition, some social workers felt that the determination of eligibility for income support should not be undertaken by professionally qualified staff. This, they believed, created an undesirable role conflict in which social workers seeking to provide help and professional advice would also have to decide whether their clients should receive material benefits. Stressing the potential harm that this conflict would cause, they urged the separation of these functions.

With the recent emphasis placed on welfare to work programs in many countries, the question of social work's involvement in these programs deserves wider discussion. Although it has already been shown that the profession has, for various reasons, been reluctant to embrace statutory income support programs, it can be argued that social workers have an important role to play in counseling and assisting clients who seek employment. This is particularly relevant in situations where people face barriers to employment arising out of the personal, familial or social challenges that social workers have traditionally sought to address. Of course, if the goal of welfare to work programs is simply to abrogate government responsibility by cutting social expenditures and reducing the caseload, the profession should not only decline to be involved but actively resist the cynical use of these programs. On the other hand, if welfare to work programs are part of a wider strategy designed to achieve the goal of eradicating poverty, social work should support these efforts by offering its expertise and engaging more effectively in these programs.

Generally, the social work literature on welfare to work programs has taken a critical stance, criticizing these programs for coercing poor people to work for low wages. Many studies, particularly in the United States, have emphasized the negative impact of welfare to work programs on children and families, and have shown that many of those who are no longer in receipt of income benefits face severe hardships. On the other hand, case studies of the effective involvement of social workers in welfare to work programs are available. Obviously, the issue needs to be more extensively debated and the social work profession needs to take a position on the role it should play in welfare to work. It is not only a question of whether social workers should engage in forms of professional practice that facilitate participation in employment for those who wish to pursue this option, but of how the profession can actively support wider social policy initiatives designed to eradicate poverty and promote social inclusion. At a time when many governments in the industrial world are retrenching social expenditures and privatizing social programs, the social work profession needs to be more actively engaged in lobbying for social and economic policies that promote social investments, maximize opportunities, foster productive employment, ensure a decent standard of living for all, and facilitate the full participation of all in the economic, political, cultural and social life of the community.

This special volume is concerned with the role of the social work profession in welfare to work programs in different countries. The book is comprised of a collection of papers presented at a symposium organized by the School of Social Welfare at the University of California, Berkeley in collaboration with the University of Bath in England, the University of Hong Kong and the University of Queensland in Australia. (One additional paper, by Hetling, Tracy and Born was not presented at the conference.) The symposium was held in April, 2005 and was the fifth in a series of international symposia hosted by the School. Organized under the topic *Social Work and Welfare to Work Programs*, the papers presented at the symposium dealt with different aspects of welfare to work and the role of social workers in these programs in the United Kingdom, Hong Kong, Australia and the United States. In addition to the formal presentation of papers, the topic was extensively discussed. The gist of these discussions is summarized at the end of this work by Professor Jane Millar of the University of Bath and Professor Michael Austin of the University of California.

The collection begins with three papers from the United States by James Midgley, Jill Duerr Berrick and her collaborators, and Andrea Hetling, Kirk Tracy and Catherine Born. After the abolition of the country's Aid to Families with Dependent Children (or AFDC) program, its replacement with a new mandatory work and time-limits program known as Temporary Assistance for Needy Families (or TANF) has attracted a great deal of international attention and is, in some circles, viewed as a model which should be emulated. Midgley offers a brief historical overview of these developments and shows that although social workers have not been at the forefront of income support and welfare to work programs, they have played a limited, and indirect role. Berrick et al.'s paper examines the role of child welfare workers involved in welfare to work programs for dually-involved clients. Reporting on her work examining several California counties implementing a coordinated service delivery model, Berrick et al. suggest the promise of social worker involvement for families challenged in fulfilling their roles both as economic providers and as parents. Hetling et al. present information on a diversion program, which provides a lump sum of cash to alleviate short-term emergencies and prevent the need for ongoing TANF receipt.

The following three papers address issues of social work and welfare to work in the United Kingdom. Martin Evans and Jane Millar outline welfare to work initiatives introduced by the Labour government since 1997 and discuss their impact on single parents. Two papers address specific fields of social work practice that interface with welfare to work programs. Nick Gould discusses social inclusion in mental health policy in the United Kingdom and asks whether recent developments offer a "new deal" for the social work profession. Mark Baldwin's paper deals with learning disabilities and focuses on the role of income support and employment in programs designed to address those challenged by these disabilities.

The next paper by Catherine McDonald and Lesley Chenoweth describes the Australian government's welfare to work program as "exceptional" and discusses the role of social workers in two agencies–the Job Network and CentreLink.

In the following paper, Kwong leung Tang reports on recent developments in Hong Kong where the government has introduced an experimental program designed to assist beneficiaries of means-tested unemployment benefits to find work. A unique feature of the program is the involvement of non-profit organizations that are contracting with the government to provide a variety of services that will facilitate the transition of unemployed adults to regular employment. Tang shows that social workers have been actively involved in this program and that they have much to contribute to the field.

The volume concludes with a short summary of the discussions arising out of the symposium by Jane Millar and Michael J. Austin. They show that the topic is pertinent to social work and its mission, and they urge the profession to engage more actively in these programs and to address systematically the issues raised by the recent policy changes that have taken place in the field of income support and welfare to work.

Welfare and Welfare to Work in the United States: The Role of Social Work

James Midgley

SUMMARY. Despite social work's historic ambivalence toward income support programs, the policy changes introduced by the TANF welfare to work program demand the profession's attention. Although social workers are not directly responsible for the administration or implementation of the program, many serve TANF clients whose lives have been affected by these changes. Tracing social work's historic but reluctant involvement with income support, this paper urges the profession to respond to the challenges posed by the TANF program in a more systematic way and to contribute more effectively to the wider task of poverty eradication. *[Article copies available for a fee from The Haworth Document Delivery Service: 1-800-HAWORTH. E-mail address: <docdelivery@haworthpress.com> Website: <http://www.HaworthPress.com> © 2006 by The Haworth Press, Inc. All rights reserved.]*

KEYWORDS. Temporary Assistance to Needy Families, TANF, welfare to work, American social policy, income support

---

James Midgley is Dean and Specht Professor, School of Social Welfare, University of California, Berkeley, 120 Haviland Hall, Berkeley, CA 94704 (E-mail: swdean@berkeley.edu).

[Haworth co-indexing entry note]: "Welfare and Welfare to Work in the United States: The Role of Social Work." Midgley, James. Co-published simultaneously in *Journal of Policy Practice* (The Haworth Press, Inc.) Vol. 5, No. 2/3, 2006, pp. 7-25; and: *International Perspectives on Welfare to Work Policy* (ed: Richard Hoefer, and James Midgley) The Haworth Press, Inc., 2006, pp. 7-25. Single or multiple copies of this article are available for a fee from The Haworth Document Delivery Service [1-800-HAWORTH, 9:00 a.m. - 5:00 p.m. (EST). E-mail address: docdelivery@ haworthpress.com].

doi:10.1300/J508v05n02_02

In the United States, the federal and state governments administer a variety of means-tested income support programs that are loosely referred to as "welfare." Between 1935 and 1996, the most important of these programs was Aid to Families with Dependent Children or AFDC. The program provided cash benefits to needy families comprised primarily of women with young children. Originally, it was expected that the beneficiaries of the program would remain at home to care for their children, but subsequently it was modified to encourage employment. Various steps were taken to enhance the educational and skill levels of welfare recipients in the hope that they would find jobs and exit the system. The first welfare to work program was introduced in the 1960s, but it was only in the 1990s that work became a policy priority. In contrast to the emphasis placed on education and training in early welfare to work programs, "work first" interventions that stress the need for immediate employment are now emphasized. Advocates of this approach believe that work should take precedence over education and job training and that welfare recipients should be required to work as a condition for receiving benefits.

In 1996, the AFDC program was replaced with Temporary Assistance for Needy Families or TANF. The new TANF program is designed to reduce the numbers as well as the length of time recipients may receive benefits by requiring them to engage in employment. Various other conditions are also imposed. Ultimately, the program seeks to shift the vast majority of recipients into regular employment. Only a small number who are deemed to be unable to work on a regular basis are exempted from the program's requirements.

Since the introduction of the TANF program, the number of welfare recipients has fallen dramatically and the program is widely regarded to have been successful. However, while a significant proportion of those who have left welfare have secured regular employment, many others work on an intermittent basis and some do not work at all. In addition, there is a good deal of evidence to show that many welfare leavers struggle to make ends meet. The hope that welfare to work would propel the beneficiaries of income support into steady productive employment and help them to enjoy a decent standard of living has not been realized.

Many people believe that the social work profession is responsible for the administration and implementation of income support and welfare to work programs, but social workers are only tangentially involved. Indeed, the profession has long had an ambivalent attitude towards income support. Although some of the profession's founders supported campaigns to expand income support programs in the early

20th century, others were critical of public poor relief. Similarly, while social workers were influential in shaping income support programs during the Roosevelt administration, relatively few social workers were subsequently employed in federal and state agencies responsible for these programs. Despite the fact that the term "social worker" was frequently used to designate staff responsible for determining the eligibility of applicants for income benefits, and ensuring that applications were processed and benefits paid, few of these staff were professionally qualified in social work.

Although, social workers today are not directly responsible for the administration of the TANF program, many are indirectly involved. For example, many social workers in the fields of child welfare and mental health serve families whose lives have been impacted by the program. Similarly, many social workers are employed in nonprofit agencies that contract with government to provide services to TANF clients. As these examples suggest, the social work profession has been affected by the program and it cannot be indifferent to the changes that have taken place. Welfare to work demands the profession's involvement, particularly with regard to advocacy and the formulation of policy alternatives that transcend the program's current preoccupation with caseload reduction.

SOCIAL WORK AND WELFARE

The term "welfare" is used to refer to a variety of statutory means-tested programs in the United States that provide cash benefits or vouchers designed to raise the incomes of poor families or to provide them with food, education, housing and other benefits. Historically, the country's means-tested income support programs originated in the poor laws that were imported from Britain during the colonial period. In the 19th century, as the number of beneficiaries receiving poor relief increased, residential facilities were more frequently used to house the indigent. The fear of incarceration served as a deterrent and, it was in this context, that charitable organizations became actively involved in providing income assistance to the poor. As is well-known, social work emerged in this milieu but, despite its formative engagement with poor relief, the payment of material benefits was not thought to be an appropriate role for the nascent profession. In addition, some of the founders of social work were critical of the poor laws, believing that they fostered pauperism and contributed to the criminality and other "social pathologies" that characterized slum communities in the rapidly expanding industrial cities (Leiby, 1978).

On the other hand, some of the profession's founders supported early 20th century campaigns to introduce what were known as Mother's Pensions. These programs were enacted by the states and provided limited income benefits primarily to widows with children or to elderly women who were unable to work (Skocpol, 1992). These efforts were part of a wider progressive social reform movement that campaigned for the introduction of European-style social insurance intended to meet the contingencies of retirement, work injury, disability and unemployment. The passage of the Social Security Act in 1935 is regarded by many as the culmination of these efforts. In addition, Title IV of this legislation replaced the widows pensions with a new program known as Aid to Dependent Children (or ADC). In 1950, it was renamed Aid to Families with Dependent Children (or AFDC). Similar in many ways to Mother's Pensions, AFDC provided means-tested cash benefits primarily to female-headed families with children. Until 1996, it was the country's core income support program and was often referred to as "welfare" even though the term included other means-tested benefits as well (Weaver, 2000).

By the 1930s, efforts to shape the new social work profession had made considerable headway. Professional schools of social work offering a graduate credential had been created at a number of prestigious universities and an association representing and accrediting these schools had been created. A professional association known as the American Association of Social Workers had also been established and, like other professional organizations, it advocated for a monopoly over certain occupational functions, set practice standards, and worked diligently to identify a set of skills, knowledge and values that would mold the profession's identity. It was in this context that long-standing disagreements about social work's role in the public sector in general, and income support in particular, intensified (Leighninger, 1987).

Despite their common middle-class origins, the founders of social work had very different social and political views. The dominant group came out of the charities and were advocates of individualized social casework. Another group associated with the settlements placed more emphasis on local community organizing. Yet another group, who also had their roots in the settlements, worked in government and pioneered efforts to establish statutory programs that would provide employment opportunities for professionally qualified social workers.

Although wider social reform efforts were generally supported, there were significant differences about how much emphasis should be given to social reform. While some took the view that the profession should be vigorously engaged in campaigns against various social evils, others cautioned that this would dilute efforts to establish a new profession that would garner recognition and respect. There were differences also about the profession's role in the public sector. While the advocates of casework were either skeptical or cautious, others believed that the creation of comprehensive statutory programs and the deployment of social workers in the public sector offered the best opportunity to address the pressing social problems of the time. Yet others were critical of the statist approach, arguing that governments invariably serve the interests of the capitalist class. They argued that social workers should engage in revolutionary action and help overthrow the system (Reisch & Andrews, 2001).

The founders of social work struggled to shape the profession by advocating for the implementation of their views in the new professional schools. It is generally agreed that the advocates of individualized social casework were the most successful. Their efforts were significantly enhanced by the adoption of psychoanalysis which offered a prestigious, conceptual basis for social work practice. Although some schools affiliated with the settlement houses opposed this approach and urged the engagement of social workers in community-based practice or the public sector, they were in the minority. Eventually, a compromise was reached and these different perspectives were all accepted as legitimate professional activities. However, it was an unsteady and unequal arrangement. Although accreditation officially recognized different forms of social work practice, casework, or clinical social work as it subsequently became known, emerged as the most desirable practice modality within the profession.

Social Workers and the New Deal

The profession was uniquely placed to influence the expansion of government social programs during the New Deal. Several influential individuals who were closely associated with social work served at the highest levels in the Roosevelt administration. Nationally known figures such as Harry Hopkins and Frances Perkins actively supported the profession and urged the employment of social work in government income support programs. Hopkins himself had served as president of the American Association of Social Workers and Perkins, who had worked at Hull House, was on close personal terms with several of the profession's leaders, particularly Grace Abbot who was head of the federal government's Children's Bureau.

Hopkins actively recruited social workers from the nonprofit sector to work in the Federal Emergency Relief Administration (FERA) and his deputy, Josephine Brown, who was also actively involved with the profession, encouraged the schools to prepare their graduates for practice in the public sector. She also arranged for FERA's staff to pursue professional degrees at schools of social work. Social workers were also represented on the Committee on Economic Security which shaped the Social Security Act. After the Act's passage, Jane Hoey, who had served under Hopkins, was appointed the first Director of the Bureau of Public Assistance which was responsible for implementing the ADC and other key income support programs. Unlike many of her social work contemporaries, Hoey actually held a professional social work credential (Stadum, 1999). Subsequently, highly-placed federal officials such as Charles Schottland and Wilbur Cohen, who were also closely associated with social work, continued to advocate for the employment of professionally qualified social workers in the federal government's income support programs.

However, efforts to engage professionally qualified social workers in these programs had limited success. Leslie Leighninger (1999) notes that a very small proportion of the staff who were employed to work directly with welfare recipients were professionally qualified. Despite efforts to recruit social workers over the years, by the 1960s, only one percent of front-line caseworkers held a professional social work degree. Although a larger proportion of supervisory staff were professionally qualified, they, too, were in a small minority. There were many reasons for this situation. There were too few professional schools of social work and they produced insufficient numbers of qualified personnel who could staff the expanding income support programs. In addition, social work graduates were not attracted to the public sector and most sought employment in the more prestigious clinics and nonprofit family counseling agencies that were so highly regarded in the profession. The profession also vigorously opposed attempts to recognize undergraduate programs in social work. Although these programs could have trained professional staff who were more likely to work in the public sector, they were shunned by the profession on the ground that undergraduate education would lower standards. The extent of opposition to these programs can be gauged by the furor that accompanied Josephine Brown's decision to fund undergraduate programs in order to train staff to work for FERA (Stadum, 1999).

Social Work and the 1962 Service Amendments

Despite the popularity of the New Deal, income support programs directed at poor women and their children never enjoyed much public support and attacks on the program increased during the 1950s. The program was frequently accused of encouraging fraud and dependency, and as more people of color successfully applied for benefits, these attacks acquired a racial character. Incidents of racial discrimination were frequently reported. Unwed mothers were also targeted. Mimi Abramovitz (1988) reports that applicants with illegitimate children were often denied benefits and that the authorities increased surveillance through, for example, unannounced late night visits to determine whether there was, in fact, a cohabiting "man in the house."

One response to this situation was the idea that professional social work services should be introduced to address illegitimacy and the personal and family problems facing welfare beneficiaries. By providing professional casework services, it was believed that social workers could solve these problems and help welfare recipients to become independent and self-sufficient. The case for specialized "rehabilitative" services of this kind came from a number of the staff and the Bureau of Public Assistance who, like Jane Hoey, the first Director, were professionally qualified social workers. They were supported by Charles Schottland, the Commissioner of Social Security. Believing that social workers would promote self-sufficiency and independence, Congress amended the Social Security Act in 1956 to encourage the states to provide services of this kind (Leighninger, 1999).

Although the 1956 initiative had minimal impact, the idea of providing professional social work services to welfare recipients gained momentum and resulted, during the Kennedy administration, in what became known as the 1962 "service amendments." Schottland's earlier efforts were now championed by Wilbur Cohen who served as an Assistant Secretary in the Department of Health, Education and Welfare. Cohen had previously been on the faculty of the School of Social Work at the University of Michigan. In addition to securing the support of a number of influential social policy experts, Cohen's efforts were endorsed by the professional social work associations, and particularly by social work educators who successfully lobbied for funds to expand social work programs and train social workers for public sector employment. A study undertaken at Columbia University recommended that 100,000 professionally qualified social workers would be needed to staff the welfare programs (Leighninger, 1999).

The 1962 legislation provided a 75% uncapped, Federal matching rate for social service programs. The legislation also provided for services to be contracted out to specialized agencies that engaged in preventive and rehabilitative work. Information and referral services were expanded and greater professional involvement in the determination of eligibility was encouraged. In 1967, during the Johnson administration, further amendments to the social services provisions of the Social Security Act were introduced. An important amendment administratively separated eligibility determination and benefits processing from social services. This decision reflected a concern that professional staff would be placed in a difficult situation if they were required to deny or restrict benefits. Another feature of this legislation was the introduction of a new welfare to work program known as the Work Incentive Program (or WIN).

Although the service amendments offered an unparalleled opportunity for social work to infuse income support with professional services, and to reshape the character of the program, this opportunity was never realized. Despite the provision of additional funds to the professional schools, the numbers of graduates who found employment in the field remained small. The old problem of graduates preferring more prestigious fields of practice had apparently not been solved by the introduction of stipends and other incentives. A disinclination towards practice with welfare recipients was also affected, as Neil Gilbert (1998) suggests, by changing attitudes. Welfare clients were increasingly viewed by social workers as victims of wider social and economic injustices and, since their problems were not caused by personal inadequacies, many believed these clients needed income benefits rather than therapeutic interventions. The growing strength of the welfare rights movement and the popularity of commentaries on social work's social control function by critics such as Frances Fox Piven and Richard Cloward (1971) also deterred many graduates from seeking employment in the field. In addition, many who were recruited, soon left. Gilbert cites several studies that reported high turnover rates in social assistance agencies. As he notes, large caseloads, omnipresent regulations and a bureaucratic culture were hardly conducive to the exercise of professional expertise.

At the same time, questions about the effectiveness of professional casework services were being raised. Critics were increasingly skeptical that the goal of addressing the behavioral problems associated with welfare dependency, and motivating clients to become self-sufficient was, in fact, being achieved. Caseloads were not declining and expenditures on social services were hardly being contained. In addition, the services provided by social workers were said to be vague and intangible. Skeptics charged that these services often amounted to little more than a pleasant conversation with clients (Gilbert, 1998). These criticisms also resulted in a sharp distinction being drawn between what were known as "soft" and "hard" services. The former involved counseling while the latter involved interventions such as day-care services, job-training, and referral to drug treatment centers (Gilbert, 1998). Not surprisingly, the latter were preferred and funds were increasingly allocated to programs of this kind. Since contracting agencies often provided "hard" services, their role expanded and although many employed social workers, they were not viewed as being a part of the public welfare system.

By the 1970s, the involvement of professional qualified social workers in income support was widely questioned, and the idea that caseloads could be reduced through professional counseling was largely discredited. As AFDC caseloads and expenditures continued to rise, politicians on the political right sought more radical solutions. President Nixon's Family Assistance Plan sought to abolish the AFDC program and replace it with a guaranteed minimum income. Bruce Jansson (2005) notes that this initiative was, in part, motivated by a desire to rid the program of social workers who, it was claimed, were responsible for its generosity and lax administration. Although this proposal was not implemented, it fostered a growing resentment towards the payment of unconditional income benefits to women with children, who were alleged to be indolent and irresponsible. The patriarchal and racist innuendos of criticisms against the program helped to pave the way for radical changes in the 1980s. In addition to retrenchment, these involved a growing emphasis on conditionality particularly with regard to work.

SOCIAL WORK AND WELFARE TO WORK PROGRAMS

By the 1980s, the hope that professionally qualified social workers would play a major role in income support programs had not been realized. Influential supporters of the profession within the federal government had retired, and they were replaced by administrators who were indifferent or even critical of social work. The service amendments had not produced the desired results and social workers were often blamed for spiraling AFDC caseloads and expenditures. One example was the criticism leveled against Mitch Ginsberg, the Commissioner for Public Welfare for New York City, who was accused of encouraging his staff to be excessively generous in determining eligibility for benefits. A social worker, Ginsberg was the former dean of the School of Social Work at Columbia University (Schmidtz & Goodin, 1998).

The Reagan administration rejected the idea that welfare recipients could be assisted to find gainful employment through professional counseling and favored a more radical approach that compelled welfare clients to work. Although it was, as Charles Murray (1984) recognized, politically unthinkable to propose that the welfare system be abolished, its expansion could be halted and even reversed. In addition to caricaturing welfare recipients and ridiculing them through gender and racial stereotypes, the administration retrenched the AFDC program. With the enactment of the Omnibus Budget and Reconciliation Act (or OBRA) in 1981, approximately 408,000 families were expelled from the welfare system and another 299,000 experienced benefit reductions. Stricter eligibility requirements were also imposed and compliance monitoring was increased (Stoesz, 2000).

Faced with a vigorous assault from the political right, Democrats were thrown into disarray and sought a compromise which would facilitate greater labor force participation among welfare recipients by emphasizing education and job training. These efforts resulted in the enactment of the Family Support Act of 1998 which required welfare recipients to participate in education and job training programs. Although many recipients were exempted from the provisions of the legislation, those who failed to participate were sanctioned either through the reduction or termination of benefits. However, the program was poorly funded and haphazardly implemented. In addition, the recession of the early 1990s increased the numbers of people receiving benefits. Accordingly, the goal of reducing the caseload through human capital investments was not realized.

There were many on the political right who were dismissive of the human capital approach. Instead, they advocated an alternative "work first" approach that requires the immediate job placement of welfare recipients irrespective of their educational level or skills. Those who fail to comply with work and other requirements should, they believe, be sanctioned. A leading advocate of this approach is Lawrence Mead (1992, 1997) who contends that the use of these "paternalistic" measures will bring about desirable behavioral changes and help welfare recipients acquire the skills they need to improve their situation and live productive lives.

In addition to promoting a work first approach, the political right's campaign for "welfare reform," as it became known, involved the devolution of income support to the states. This was the declared goal of the

Reagan administration's "New Federalism" which had replaced various federal entitlement programs with block grant funding. In the 1980s, no less than 57 federal health and social services programs were merged into nine block grants that the states could use to fund maternal and child health services, services for the mentally ill and community development programs. The social services program, which was originally intended to provide professional counseling to welfare recipients, was also block granted. In addition, it was significantly retrenched, and the funding provided to schools of social work to train professionals for employment in the public social services was terminated (Reisch, 1995).

However, it did not prove politically possible at the time to devolve the AFDC program to the states. Instead, the Reagan administration set into motion a process of granting waivers that permitted the states to experiment with a variety of innovations designed to change the attitudes and behaviors of welfare recipients, and compel them to work. New phrases such as "learnfare" and "workfare" now entered the welfare vocabulary. These terms connoted experimental programs that required welfare recipients to participate in municipal public works programs or to ensure that their children attend school regularly. These waivers gathered momentum and, by the early 1990s, the scene had been set for the devolution of the AFDC program.

When the Republican Party gained a majority in Congress in 1994, the proponents of welfare reform redoubled their efforts to devolve the AFDC program and to restructure it by imposing strict work requirements on welfare recipients. Challenging President Bill Clinton to fulfill his promise to "end welfare as we know it," they redrafted his original welfare reform legislation and, in 1996, secured passage of the Personal Responsibility and Work Opportunity Reconciliation Act. This legislation created the TANF program. In keeping with the Republican commitment to devolution, it ended the "entitlement" provision of AFDC, and the states were now given a fixed federal allocation in the form of a block grant.

Various conditionality requirements were also imposed, abrogating the notion that claimants had a "social right" to receive assistance. The states were required to ensure that recipients engaged in employment, and goals for labor force participation were set. Time limits that restricted the payment of benefits to a lifetime maximum of 60 months were also imposed. However, the legislation allowed 20% of the caseload to be exempted from the requirement. Sanctions that ensured that welfare recipients conformed to the demands of the TANF program were also featured prominently. Although the program imposed conditionality requirements, non-punitive provisions were also introduced. An important innovation was the Child Care and Development Fund which allocated additional resources for day care. The asset and income restrictions of the AFDC program were also relaxed to permit recipients to own a motor car and other assets and still receive benefits. Other policies and programs introduced by the Clinton administration also softened the provisions of the legislation. For example, an increase in the minimum wage and the Earned Income Tax Credit have furthered the goal of "making work pay." In addition, with the passage of the Workforce Investment Act of 1998, a plethora of poorly coordinated job training, literacy and adult education programs were consolidated, and opportunities for welfare recipients to find regular employment were enhanced.

The Social Effects of the TANF Program

Both Republicans and Democrats have claimed that the TANF program has been a huge success and both parties, and their leaders, have taken credit for introducing the program. Statistical data show that there has indeed been a substantial decline in the numbers receiving benefits and many believe that a dramatic shift from dependency to self-sufficiency has taken place. Weaver (2000) reports that the numbers receiving income support declined by about 51%–from about 14.2 million in 1994 to about 6.9 million in 1999. Besharov and Germanis (2003) reveal that by 2001, further declines had been recorded amounting to a total caseload reduction of about 59% or nine million individuals.

Although these trends seem to support the view that the aggressive imposition of work requirements ends welfare dependency and facilitates the transition of welfare recipients into steady employment and a decent standard of living, a number of studies that have tracked those who have left welfare questions this contention. These "leaver studies" as they are known, reveal that while the majority indeed reported that they were working, only a minority was employed in permanent, regular jobs. In one long-term study undertaken in the state of Washington, most leavers reported working an average of 34 out of the preceding 52 weeks (Brauner & Loprest, 1999). Besharov and Germanis (2000) estimated that as many as 40% of leavers were working intermittently and relying on support from partners, family members and friends as well as other sources of government assistance such as food stamps. Loprest (1999) found that 20% reported no work activity and no income from a partner or other form of government aid. A subsequent review of 15 leaver studies confirmed these findings (Acs & Loprest, 2004). In 2002, about 40% of leavers had steady, regular jobs while about 30% worked intermittently. The remainder (30%) reported no work activity. In addition, most worked for low wages.

The argument that the imposition of work requirements will propel welfare recipients into sustained, productive employment is also countered by studies that reveal that a significant number of those who left the TANF program return to claim benefits again. In Wisconsin, where the program is reputed to be particularly effective, 30% of leavers returned to claim benefits within 15 months (US General Accounting Office, 1999). In her nationwide review, Pamela Loprest (1999) found that about 30% of leavers returned to the rolls, and in a subsequent study of trends in 2002, about a quarter of leavers had returned (Acs & Loprest, 2004). These findings are consistent with earlier research into welfare spells which showed that a significant proportion of those who leave welfare require assistance again (Bane & Ellwood, 1994).

The studies also show that many leavers are engaged in low-paying service occupations. Several report that most leavers had incomes that were only marginally above the poverty line (Brauner & Loprest, 1999; Acs & Loprest, 2004). While it is true that their incomes are augmented by the Earned Income Tax Credit, child support payments and other sources, the conclusion that former welfare recipients are now self-sufficient is not supported by the evidence. In addition, the studies reveal that many welfare leavers have difficulty meeting their needs. One third reported skipping meals or reducing food intake because of insufficient incomes. More than 38% reported that they had difficulty in paying rents and utility bills. Indeed, many had defaulted on rent and utility payments since leaving welfare (Loprest, 1999; US General Accounting Office, 1999). These findings have led even some optimistic supporters of welfare reform such as Besharov and Germanis (2000, 33) to conclude that while welfare reform has not been a social catastrophe as liberals had predicted, "neither has it lifted large numbers of female headed households out of poverty."

These studies refer only to those who have left the welfare system and it is, of course, true that many of those who remain in the system participate in work activities while continuing to receive benefits. While this would appear to be preferable to being wholly dependent on benefits, research into those who remain in the program also questions the assumption that standards of living among current welfare recipients have improved significantly as a result of the imposition of work requirements. An official government study revealed that 13% of clients reported falling behind with rent payments, 16% did not meet utility bills, 11% could not afford child care and 6% experienced times when they could not afford food (US General Accounting Office, 1999).

These findings confirm earlier studies that showed how difficult it is for welfare recipients to make ends meet. Indeed, ethnographic research undertaken before the introduction of the TANF program found that most of those receiving AFDC benefits were illicitly engaged in intermittent and low-paid employment in order to secure a minimum standard of living (Edin & Lein, 1997; Harris, 1993; Harris, 1997). Welfare benefits were viewed as just one of various sources of boosting household income. In addition to illicit employment, incomes were augmented with child support payments, gifts, loans and in-kind assistance from parents and friends. This finding also questions the claim that welfare reform has indeed shifted a large number of welfare recipients from being economically inactive and dependent on welfare, to being regularly employed and self-sufficient. Many who were believed to be economically inactive were, in fact, engaged in various forms of clandestine employment and self-employment but at income levels that were too low to raise them much above the poverty level. Research into the effects of welfare reform suggest that many who are no longer on welfare, as well as those who are still receiving benefits, continue to cope as best they can by engaging in low-paid employment on the margins of the economy.

CHALLENGES FOR SOCIAL WORK

The replacement of the AFDC income support program by the TANF welfare to work program has indeed achieved the goal of reducing the caseload and cutting social assistance expenditures. But there is little evidence to show that the program has propelled many former welfare recipients into regular, productive employment or provided them with the opportunity to realize the promise of securing a comfortable standard of living through individual effort and hard work. Of course, there are exceptions and case study material is available to show that some former welfare recipients have indeed benefited from education, training and job placement programs. But, as the research cited earlier reveals, many poor people who previously increased their incomes through receiving income support benefits are still poor and are still struggling to make ends meet.

This finding has obvious implications for the social work profession. Although social workers have not played a significant role in the administration and implementation of income support programs, they have historically been engaged with poor people and have frequently worked with clients who received benefits. Many of the child welfare, mental health, substance abuse and other problems they deal with are concentrated among poor families. The research studies cited earlier reveal that the problems of material deprivation facing the profession's clients have not been resolved by the termination or reduction of income support. These problems are particularly challenging for those who have been sanctioned. Many sanctioned clients are categorized as "hard to serve," and they face exceptional hardships as a result of inadequate educational and personal skills, medical and mental health problems and substance abuse. Several studies have shown that the challenges facing these clients are so severe that few are able to function independently outside the welfare system (Marcenko & Fagan, 1996) and that sanctions do little to produce the changes predicted by the advocates of welfare paternalism (Lindhorst, Mancoske, & Kemp, 2000; Ong & Houston, 2005; Reichman, Teitler, & Curtis, 2005). These challenges also have negative effects on children and it is not surprising that many social workers who serve welfare recipients are also involved in the statutory child welfare system.

Although it would seem obvious that the challenges facing these clients and their families demand professional social work intervention, social workers are not directly employed in the TANF program to help these clients. Instead, those with special needs may be referred to specialized agencies, or otherwise, these agencies may encounter these clients without any referral. This haphazard system has resulted in the fragmentation of services and in poor coordination between different agencies working with the same family. The traditional separation of the statutory child welfare and income support systems has long been viewed as a problem by social workers. Many believe that efforts to deal with child neglect and abuse and with the problems children encounter in schools, cannot be separated from the problem of material deprivation which the income support system is supposed to address. This is hardly a new issue. Indeed, it was an important consideration when the service amendments of 1962 were being debated.

Although there is an obvious need to more effectively coordinate these services, it appears that officials administering the TANF program and social workers in public child welfare, mental health, and substance abuse programs do not collaborate closely. This is also the case with social workers in nonprofit agencies that contract with statutory agencies to serve TANF clients. It might be expected that these agencies will work closely with government officials responsible for administering the TANF program, but this is questionable. Indeed, a rather depressing study of senior social work staff at 107 nonprofit agencies that provide service to TANF clients in New York (Abramovitz, 2005) found that these agencies face a number of serious challenges which impede collaboration and effective service delivery.

These challenges, as well as the needs of both those who have left and those who continue on the TANF program, demand the profession's attention. The profession's historic disinclination to engage directly with issues of income support, and with the wider problems of poverty and deprivation, should be reversed. Although some social workers have claimed that the issue of material need is beyond their purview, the stark realities of poverty and material need that characterize the lives of so many clients cannot be ignored. Although belated, the profession needs to engage the welfare to work system in a much more systematic way. Closer links between social workers and officials administering and implementing the TANF program need to be forged. Coordination of services needs to be strengthened and efforts to mitigate the hardships of sanctions on clients should be redoubled. This will require more than the efforts of individual social workers and administrators. Professional social work associations need to recognize that they have been marginal to the dramatic policy shifts that have taken place in recent years and they need to make a concerted effort to support practitioners in both the public and nonprofit sectors who engage the welfare to work system.

The challenges of the TANF welfare to work program have obvious implications for social work education. Schools of social work need to pay more attention to the issues raised by the emphasis that has now been placed on welfare to work. Instead of merely criticizing or even dismissing these programs, the challenges the new system poses for everyday social work practice should be recognized. If social work students fully understand the complex issues welfare to work programs raise for their clients, they will be better prepared to address them.

In addition to developing strategies for better accommodating social work practice with the realities of welfare to work, the social work profession needs to embark more vigorously on initiatives that mitigate its negative effects. Examples of innovative initiatives that seek to find opportunities for utilizing the TANF program in positive ways can be given. For example, social workers have been actively involved in community-based projects that support local micro enterprises (Banerjee, 2001; Straatmann, & Sherraden, 2001), promote local community work force development initiatives (Shivula & Austin, 2001) and develop partnerships between local nonprofit organizations serving TANF clients (Libby & Austin, 2004). Social workers also have a vital role to play in helping clients secure access to the services to which they are entitled. The TANF program's disincentive effects have led many clients to believe that they no longer qualify for food stamps, child-care subsidies, housing assistance and other means-tested benefits, and accordingly, the numbers receiving these benefits have also fallen. In addition to encouraging their clients to apply for these benefits, a special effort needs to be made to advise them of their rights to qualify for the Earned Income Tax Credit which subsidizes the incomes of poor working families but which is still not fully utilized by these families.

The profession also needs to step up its lobbying efforts to question the assumptions on which the TANF program is based, and challenge its current emphasis on caseload reduction. Collaboration with other professional associations and organizations that are campaigning for the reform of the system should be increased. There is potential for working more closely with child welfare advocacy organizations to protect children affected by the program, and particularly with faith-based organizations concerned with these issues. Greater efforts are also needed to build coalitions with conservatives who believe that government has a role to play in ensuring the welfare of families and children. The profession should also support efforts to identify new approaches that offer a viable alternative to the punitive approach of the TANF program. New ideas that can provide a basis for political action are urgently needed. The ideological hegemony of marketism, traditionalism and regulationism in American political and social life can only be challenged by the formulation of vibrant, new ideas that offer viable alternatives. The persistence of poverty in the context of so much affluence demands action and the social work profession needs to respond more systematically to the challenge of eradicating poverty from American society.

REFERENCES

Abramovitz, M. (1988). *Regulating the Lives of Women: Social Welfare Policy from Colonial Times to the Present*. Boston: South End Press.

Abramovitz, M. (2005). The largely untold story of welfare reform and the human services. *Social Work, 50*(2), 175-186.

Acs, G., & Loprest, P. (2004). *Leaving Welfare: Employment and Well-Being of Families That Left Welfare in the Post-Entitlement Era.* Kalamazoo, MI: W.E. Upjohn Institute.

Bane, M. J., & Ellwood, D. T. (1994). *Welfare Realities: From Rhetoric to Reform.* Cambridge, MA: Harvard University Press.

Banerjee, M. M. (2001). Micro-enterprise training (MET) program: An innovative response to welfare reform. *Journal of Community Practice, 9*(3), 87-107.

Besharov, D. J., & Germanis, P. (2000). Welfare reform: Four years later. *The Public Interest, 140,* 17-35.

Besharov, D. J., & Germanis, P. (2003). Welfare reform and the caseload decline. In D. Besharov (Ed.), *Family and Child Well-Being After Welfare Reform.* New Brunswick, NJ: Transaction Publishers, pp. 35-66.

Brauner, S., & Loprest, P. (1999). *Where Are They Now? What State Studies of People Who Left Welfare Tell Us.* Washington, DC: The Urban Institute.

Edin, K., & Lein, L. (1997). *Making Ends Meet: How Single Mothers Survive Welfare and Low Wage Work.* New York: Russell Sage Foundation.

Gilbert, N. (1998). From service to social control: Implications of welfare reform for professional practice in the United States. *European Journal of Social Work, 1*(1), 101-108.

Harris, K. M. (1993). Work and welfare among single mothers in poverty. *American Journal of Sociology, 93,* 317-352.

Harris, K. M. (1997). *Teen Mothers and the Revolving Welfare Door.* Philadelphia, PA: Temple University Press.

Jansson, B. (2005). *The Reluctant Welfare State: A History of American Social Welfare Policies.* Pacific Grove, CA: Brooks/Cole.

Leiby, J. (1978). *A History of Social Welfare and Social Work in the United States.* New York: Columbia University Press.

Leighninger, L. (1987). *Social Work: Search for Identity.* New York: Greenwood Press.

Leighninger, L. (1999). The service trap: Social work and public welfare policy in the 1960s. In G. R. Lowe & N. P. Reid (Eds.), *The Professionalization of Poverty: Social Work and the Poor in the Twentieth Century.* New York: Aldyne de Gruyter, pp. 63-88.

Libby, M. K., & Austin, M. J. (2004). Building a coalition of non-profit agencies to collaborate with a county health and human services agency. In M. J. Austin (Ed.), *Changing Welfare Services: Case Studies of Local Welfare Reform Programs.* New York: The Haworth Press, Inc., pp. 231-250.

Lindhorst, T., Mancoske, R. J., & Kemp, A. A. (2000). Is welfare reform working? A study of the effects of sanctions on families receiving Temporary Assistance to Needy Families. *Journal of Sociology and Social Welfare, 27*(4), 185-201.

Loprest, P. (1999). *How Families that Left Welfare Are Doing: A National Picture.* Washington, DC: The Urban Institute.

Marcenko, M. O., & Fagan, J. (1996). Welfare to work: What are the obstacles? *Journal of Sociology and Social Welfare, 23*(3), 111-131.

Mead, L. M. (1992). *The New Politics of Poverty: The Nonworking Poor in America.* New York: Basic Books.

Mead, L. (Ed.) (1997). *The New Paternalism: Supervisory Approaches to Poverty.* Washington, DC: Brookings Institution Press.

Murray, C. (1984). *Losing Ground: American Social Policy, 1950-1980.* New York: Basic Books.

Ong, P. M., & Houston, D. (2005). CalWorks Sanction Patterns in Four Counties: An Analysis of Administrative Data. Berkeley, CA: California Policy Research Center, University of California.

Piven, F. F., & Cloward, R. A. (1971). *Regulating the Poor: The Functions of Public Welfare.* New York: Pantheon.

Reichman, N. E., Teitler, J. O., & Curtis, M. A. (2005). TANF sanctions and hardship. *Social Service Review, 79*(2), 215-236.

Reisch, M. (1995). Public social services. In R. Edwards (Ed.), *Encyclopedia of Social Work,* 19th edition. Washington, DC: NASW Press.

Reisch, M., & Andrews, J. (2001). *The Road Not Taken: A History of Radical Social Work in the United States.* Philadelphia, PA: Brunner-Routledge.

Schmidtz, D., & Goodin, R. E. (1998). *Social Welfare and Individual Responsibility.* New York: Cambridge University Press.

Shivula, J., & Austin, M. J. (2004). Fostering neighborhood involvement in workforce development: The Alameda County Neighborhood Jobs Pilot Program. In M.J. Austin (Ed.), *Changing Welfare Services: Case Studies of Local Welfare Reform Programs.* New York: The Haworth Press, Inc., pp. 189-216.

Skocpol, T. (1992). *Protecting Soldiers and Mothers: The Political Origins of Social Policy in the United States.* Cambridge, MA: Harvard University Press.

Stadum, B. (1999). The uneasy marriage of professional social work and public relief, 1870-1940. In G.R. Lowe & N.P. Reid (Eds.), *The Professionalization of Poverty: Social Work and the Poor in the Twentieth Century.* New York: Aldyne de Gruyter.

Stoesz, D. (2000). Social policy: Reagan and beyond. In J. Midgley, M. B. Tracy, & M. Livermore (Eds.), *Handbook of Social Policy.* Thousand Oaks, CA: Sage Publications, pp. 143-153.

Straatmann, S., & Sherraden, M. (2001). Welfare to self-employment: A case study of the First Step Fund. *Journal of Community Practice, 9*(3): 73-94.

US General Accounting Office (1999). *Welfare Reform: Information on Former Recipients' Status.* Washington, DC.

Weaver, R. K. (2000). *Ending Welfare as We Know it.* Washington, DC: Brookings.

Wenocur, S., & Reisch, M. (1989). *From Charity to Enterprise: The Development of American Social Work in a Market Economy.* Urbana, IL: University of Illinois Press.

Working Together
for Children and Families:
Where TANF and Child Welfare Meet

Jill Duerr Berrick
Laura Frame
Jodie Langs
Lisa Varchol

SUMMARY. While the organizational systems designed to provide cash assistance and child welfare services have been separate since the 1970s, changes wrought by welfare reform in the late 1990s suggest new opportunities for organizational collaboration. This paper examines the link between family poverty and child maltreatment, and the policy levers that can be employed to inhibit or promote child and family well-

---

Jill Duerr Berrick, PhD, is Associate Professor, University of California, Berkeley, School of Social Welfare, 120 Haviland Hall, Berkeley, CA 94704 (E-mail: dberrick@ berkeley.edu). Laura Frame, PhD, is a former researcher at the Center for Social Services Research, and is affiliated with Children's Hospital and Research Center, Oakland, CA. Jodie Langs received her MSW in 2004 from UC Berkeley (E-mail: Jodielangs@yahoo.com). Lisa Varchol received her MSW in 2005 from UC Berkeley (E-mail: lisavar@aol.com).

The authors thank Anne Geiger and Stephanie Cosner Berzin for their assistance. Special thanks to Kate Karpilow and Linda Orrante for their enthusiasm and creativity in bringing integrated services to California, and to the staff of the 13 counties who gave their time to share insights about program collaboration.

[Haworth co-indexing entry note]: "Working Together for Children and Families: Where TANF and Child Welfare Meet." Berrick, Jill Duerr et al. Co-published simultaneously in *Journal of Policy Practice* (The Haworth Press, Inc.) Vol. 5, No. 2/3, 2006, pp. 27-42; and: *International Perspectives on Welfare to Work Policy* (ed: Richard Hoefer, and James Midgley) The Haworth Press, Inc., 2006, pp. 27-42. Single or multiple copies of this article are available for a fee from The Haworth Document Delivery Service [1-800- HAWORTH, 9:00 a.m. - 5:00 p.m. (EST). E-mail address: docdelivery@ haworthpress.com].

being within the context of welfare reform. It then reviews one state's experience with inter-organizational collaboration between welfare and child welfare and the special challenges agencies face in attempting to streamline services. *[Article copies available for a fee from The Haworth Document Delivery Service: 1-800-HAWORTH. E-mail address: <docdelivery@ haworthpress.com> Website: <http://www.HaworthPress.com> © 2006 by The Haworth Press, Inc. All rights reserved.]*

KEYWORDS. TANF, child welfare, welfare reform

Temporary Assistance to Needy Families is designed to offer cash assistance to low-income families, the majority of whom are headed by single mothers. In general, typical service activities of TANF staff focus on accessing employment-related information for clients, assessing and addressing barriers to employment, and offering services to propel and support movement into the labor market (Nightingale, Kramer, Trutko, Egner, & Barnow, 2003; Thompson, Van Nexx, & O'Brien, 2001). Child welfare services are designed to support parents in their parenting role and protect children from maltreatment. Typical service activities of child welfare staff center on assessing child safety, determining family problems and needs, and accessing resources to support parents and reduce the likelihood of maltreatment recurrence (Ginsberg, 2001). While the goals of these programs differ, they share a great deal in common. Both programs target families struggling to get by in one or more life domains; they also largely serve very young children. Two-thirds of clients involved in TANF are children, and half of these are ages six or younger (U.S. House of Representatives, 2004). Of the cases reported to child welfare services, the youngest among these are the most likely to be victimized (USDHHS, 2005). Both programs are aimed at assisting parents in their roles vis-à-vis children: TANF focuses on the parent's role as a provider, and child welfare focuses on the parent's role as a caregiver. In many cases, both programs also target–largely or entirely–populations struggling with the challenges posed by American poverty.

While the organizational systems designed to provide cash assistance and child welfare services have been separate since the 1970s (see Frame, 1999 for a review), changes wrought by welfare reform in the late 1990s suggest new opportunities for organizational collaboration. What are the links between family poverty and child maltreatment, and to what extent will TANF propel greater numbers of vulnerable families into the child welfare system? After reviewing these questions, this paper examines one state's experience with inter-organizational collaboration between welfare and child welfare services.

THE INTERSECT: POVERTY AND MALTREATMENT

Research has demonstrated a strong correlation between poverty and child maltreatment. For example, the Third National Incidence Study of Child Abuse and Neglect (NIS-3) revealed that children from families with incomes below $15,000 were more than 20 times more likely to be maltreated than children from homes where family income was greater than $30,000 (Sedlak & Broadhurst, 1996). Although poverty is the strongest predictor of maltreatment, the correlation between the two phenomena does not signify causation. Instead, a confluence of factors related to poverty appear to exert certain pressures on parenting such as parental stress precipitated by material hardship, and other stressful life events that, in turn, can detrimentally affect parenting behaviors (Berger & Brooks-Gunn, 2005). Thus, TANF policies may serve to increase the likelihood of child welfare involvement for poor families if policies such as work requirements, sanctions, and lifetime limits reduce the material resources available to families and heighten the experience of parental stress. Conversely, policies may serve to reduce maltreatment rates if child poverty rates are decreased, and factors such as parental stress are ameliorated (Frame & Berrick, 2003). Before welfare reform, researchers knew little about the relationship between family involvement in welfare and the family's subsequent or simultaneous involvement in the child welfare program. Since the late 1990s, research in this area has expanded substantially.

Welfare and Child Welfare Populations

Though poverty is a predictor of child maltreatment, the majority of those who receive welfare assistance do not maltreat their children. To gain an understanding about the scope of the overlap, it is useful to consider, relative to the general population, the extent to which the population of children in poverty intersects with the population of those children who are also involved with child welfare services. As of the last census count, there were approximately 72.6 million children under the age of 18 in the United States. The proportion of children in poverty was 16.3% of the child population, or 11.8 million children. The child welfare population is significantly smaller than the child poverty population. In 2002, it is estimated that there were 896,000 victims of child abuse or neglect in the U.S. Of these, approximately 20% (about 196,000) were placed in out-of-home care (U.S.D.H.H.S., 2002). It is estimated that a majority of the children affected by child maltreatment come from the child poverty population (Geen & Tumlin, 1999). Figure 1 graphically displays the overlap of the child welfare and welfare populations.

Given that only a relatively modest proportion of families receiving welfare also have child welfare involvement, it is helpful to review the factors and characteristics, in addition to socioeconomic disadvantage, that are associated with child abuse and neglect.

Characteristics of Families Dually Involved in TANF and Child Welfare

Using pre-TANF data, several studies have examined the characteristics of welfare recipients that are associated with increased likelihood of a child welfare event. Using linked administrative data, Needell et al. (1999) examined a cohort of 63,768 children in 10 California counties entering

FIGURE 1. Proportion of Children in Foster Care as Compared to Those in Poverty in the U.S. (not to scale)

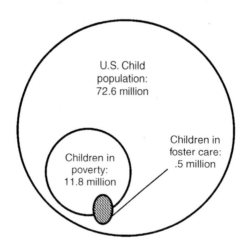

U.S. Child population: 72.6 million

Children in foster care: .5 million

Children in poverty: 11.8 million

AFDC for the first time between 1990 and 1995. When the researchers examined child welfare involvement for the 1990 cohort, Needell and co-authors found that 27% of the 1990 entrants had a maltreatment report during the five-year study period. Beyond the reporting stage, 8% had an open case, and 3% of the entry cohort was placed into foster care. Further examination of the characteristics of child AFDC entrants with child welfare contact indicates that certain factors are associated with increased odds of a child welfare event. Specifically, infants, children from single-parent households, those with late or no prenatal care, Caucasian children, children born with low birthweight, and those born into large families had an increased risk, relative to their counterparts, of experiencing a child welfare event. Furthermore, increased time on aid and breaks in aid receipt (both AFDC and Medicaid) were associated with a higher likelihood of experiencing a child welfare event. These findings point to vulnerabilities among the welfare population that may serve as a preliminary means to targeted interventions.

In addition to child- and family-level demographic variables associated with increased risk for child maltreatment among welfare recipients, other studies have examined the role of variables associated with financial stress. For example, in a study examining the relationship between welfare grant reductions (including sanctions) and child welfare involvement among a random sample of 706 Chicago AFDC recipients in 1995 and 1996, Shook (1999) also surveyed a subsample of study participants (n = 173) to provide a more in-depth analysis of the experiences associated with changes in income among this population. The risk of child welfare involvement was significantly increased among those who experienced a grant reduction with no increase in employment income. Environmental hardships such as food or diaper shortages, an eviction threat, or utility shut-off also played a mediating role between grant reduction without subsequent employment and child welfare system involvement. Additionally, recent stressful life events such as a housing move, major household expense, or illness among a household member, compounded the risk of a child welfare event.

Courtney, Piliavin and Power (2001) examined predictors of child welfare involvement for 457 TANF applicants in Milwaukee County, both before and after TANF application. Using case-level administrative data and survey data, Courtney and his colleagues report findings consistent with those above. Namely, a greater number of children in the family and parental stress were significant predictors of child welfare involvement. Previous child protective services (CPS) investigation prior to TANF application was the best predictor of child welfare involvement. Risk of child welfare involvement was decreased for those who were currently working or had worked within the past year.

Other studies have also identified substance abuse (Courtney, Piliavin, Dworsky, & Zinn, 2001), domestic violence and a history of childhood abuse (Derr & Taylor, 2004) as factors leading to increased involvement with child welfare services among welfare recipients. In sum, studies to date suggest that a combination of child and family level characteristics, source and amount of income and economic hardships play a role in increasing the risk for child welfare involvement among families receiving public assistance. If factors associated with increasing risk for child welfare involvement are known, states can fashion their TANF programs either to increase or inhibit the risk of maltreatment among public assistance recipients.

Aspects of TANF that May Inhibit Child Safety

Increased economic hardship is correlated with an increase in the odds of a child welfare event. Accordingly, policies that result in families having fewer material resources available may result in a heightened risk of a child welfare event, particularly when combined with the stressors mentioned previously. Using state-level administrative data, findings from a series of studies by Paxson and Waldfogel (1999, 2001) may support this hypothesis. The co-authors found that full family sanctions are associated with an increase in substantiated cases of maltreatment and physical abuse. States that implemented full family sanctions experienced a 21% increase in the number of substantiated cases of maltreatment following the 1996 federal reforms (Paxson & Waldfogel, 1999). Other strict sanctions are also associated with an increase in out-of-home care. This is consistent with findings from Ovwhigo, Leavitt, and Born (2003) who found that, among families who left TANF, cases closed due to sanctions were at a higher risk of having a post-exit child welfare event than those cases closed voluntarily, due to work, or no reapplication.

The effects of TANF time limits of less than 60 months may also be associated with a large increase in substantiated maltreatment in general, and physical abuse, in particular. Paxson and Waldfogel (1999, 2001) found that the family cap policy was associated with lower maltreatment rates, but a rise in out-of-home care placements. In short, aspects of TANF that serve to decrease the resources available to families are associated with increases in maltreatment and placement in out-of-home care. These findings are consistent with those of Shook (1999) and Needell et al. (1999), which indicate that when benefits are reduced or interrupted, there is a significant increase in the odds of a child welfare event.

Waldfogel (2004) cautions that while these collective findings give cause for concern, there is still a great deal that is unknown about the effects of TANF on child welfare due to the timing of its implementation. Pre-dating PRWORA, states experimented with welfare policy through federal waivers beginning in the early 1990s. Even after the passage of the 1996 welfare reform legislation, TANF was not fully implemented in some states until later in the decade, thus limiting the strength of some of these early findings. Due to the flexibility of TANF, there is also considerable variation in the nature of the programs and policies that states have elected to implement. As a rough analysis of the impact of individual components of TANF policy on foster care caseloads, Waldfogel (2004) used "policy clusters" that measure strict vs. lenient welfare policies to assess changes in foster care caseloads from 1998-2000 across states. Her preliminary findings suggest an association between "lenient" time limit states and lower child welfare caseloads, and "strict" time limit states and increased caseloads. Future models examining a longer time span will necessarily attend to other demographic and socioeconomic factors also likely to contribute to caseload change (Waldfogel, 2004).

Aspects of TANF that May Promote Child Safety

While a reduction in family income can have negative impacts on child welfare involvement, the opposite may also be true. Namely, Paxson and Waldfogel (2001) found that states with more generous welfare benefits had lower levels of neglect and fewer children placed in out-of-home care. There were large effects associated with these results: a 10% increase in benefit levels was predicted to reduce neglect by 32%, and out-of-home care placements by 8%. The findings from Shook (1999) and Needell et al. (1999) echo the importance of welfare policies that decrease economic hardship. Specifically, when parents experience uninterrupted benefits and benefits that remain intact, risk of child welfare involvement is lowered. A study of pre-TANF families in Cuyahoga County, Ohio suggests that welfare benefits continue to matter once children are placed in out-of-home care. Wells and Guo (2003) found that, regardless of work status, children reunified more quickly when welfare benefits are consistent. Under TANF, states may choose to maintain benefits for families for six months when children enter out-of-home care. The findings by Wells and Guo suggest that states that opt into this provision may promote more timely reunification.

Employment and Maltreatment

Whereas the effects of some TANF policies on child welfare outcomes appear consistent across studies, the collective findings related to parental employment are less clear. Some studies have found that the shift from cash assistance to employment has led to an increase in child welfare involvement–particularly for child neglect–and longer lengths of stay in out-of-home care (Fein & Lee, 2000; Geen, Fender, Leos-Urbel, & Markowitz, 2001; Paxson & Waldfogel, 2001; Wells & Guo, 2004).

In contrast, other studies have noted the protective effects of parental employment in regard to child welfare. In a study examining child protection reports for TANF grantees in Illinois, Slack, Holl, Lee, McDaniel, Altenbernd and Stevens (2003) found that child welfare risk was greatest for those who continued to receive welfare with no involvement in the work force. Similarly, Courtney and colleagues (2001) found that, among TANF applicants, employment was associated with decreased risk for child welfare services involvement. Finally, Shook (1999) found that, among those who experienced a reduction in benefits, child welfare involvement was more likely for those who had no subsequent income from employment than those who had income from wages.

In short, our understanding of the relationship between parental employment and child maltreatment among welfare and former welfare recipients is obfuscated by several factors. Employment may be less relevant than the type of employment, whether work serves to increase or decrease income or other stressors, whether it is attached to other work-related benefits, and/or its effects on parents' mental health and self-esteem.

Based on the mixed findings related to parental employment and child welfare, it appears that state TANF policies that balance work force involvement with continued financial and other supportive assistance may be promising. Additionally, available research suggests that addressing barriers to work through supportive services may also serve to improve parenting. For example, if parental mental health problems are the cause of unstable employment and increased stress, providing mental health counseling or other related services may effectively decrease parental stress and enable the parent to maintain stable employment. Using TANF funds to provide supportive services could act as a child welfare intervention in that the primary risk factors associated with child maltreatment for the welfare population, namely parental stress and economic hardship, could be alleviated through a combination of benefits and supportive services.

THE PROMISE AND CHALLENGE
OF TANF/CHILD WELFARE INTEGRATION

TANF policy goals are largely associated with the movement from cash assistance to work. Under PRWORA, welfare programs were largely restructured to include an array of supportive services offered to parents to promote their ability to work. Services such as domestic violence counseling, substance abuse treatment, mental health services and child care are available to clients to the extent that these barriers prevent them from securing stable employment. As Courtney (2001) points out, these are many of the same services that are provided to parents involved with the child welfare system with the goal of improving parent functioning. This overlap points to an intersection between welfare and child welfare services that could be streamlined to address both child safety and employment goals if the two systems could sufficiently coordinate efforts to address the common barriers faced by parents.

While TANF services and supports could be utilized to help promote positive parenting among families at-risk for child welfare involvement, the knowledge-base in the child welfare system regarding risk factors for maltreatment could also be employed effectively within the larger TANF population to help determine family needs. This is not to suggest that instituting practices to monitor TANF recipients' behavior is desirable. Rather, through a comprehensive assessment, determining means to reasonably alleviate family stress within the context of resources available through TANF could prevent future negative events, such as sanctions for non-compliance, that only further pose a risk for child welfare involvement. In short, the flexibility associated with TANF legislation allows for creatively blending child welfare and TANF resources in a manner that could increase family income and improve family functioning. Under TANF, it appears that the well-being of the nation's most fragile children and families depends upon the ability of states and localities to attend to the complex barriers associated with unstable employment and parental hardship.

If TANF can be used to support positive parenting, then a restructuring of traditional services is in order to provide new services and/or a new service delivery model to TANF clients. Similarly, if child welfare staff can more effectively account for the role of poverty in increasing risk for child maltreatment and parenting challenges, efforts to make connections with TANF cash assistance programs could help to increase family income in some cases, thereby reducing the stress that accompanies parenting in poverty. One needn't look far into the TANF or the child welfare caseloads to locate families who might benefit from integrated services (see Frame & Berrick, 2003). System and service integration between TANF and child welfare bureaucracies holds promise for delivering more targeted services to families in need and– possibly–improving outcomes for poor children and families.

Opportunities for Social Work Intervention with Dually-Involved Clients

Since 2000, 13 California county administrators have experimented with child welfare/TANF collaboration under a specially designed initiative called "Linkages." Linkages included an effort to coordinate services and integrate systems between CalWORKs (California Work Opportunity and Responsibility to Kids–California's welfare to work program) and child welfare. Program administrators' goals focused on increasing client self-sufficiency; improving the relevance and quality of services to families; reducing conflicting client requirements in their interactions with the two systems; and creating safety and permanency for children.

One of the principal characteristics distinguishing Linkages from many other pilot initiatives in California and elsewhere was the role of an outside non-profit agency in facilitating the change process within counties. With financial support from a local foundation, the California Center for Research on Women and Families (CCRWF) offered modest funding to counties to initiate and maintain activities associated with the project. They organized several in-person and telephone meetings, enabling county representatives to share ideas and learn from one another; and they served as a liaison between county and state agencies. In addition, CCRWF developed a number of useful tools to assist counties in initiating and sustaining the project; to reduce redundancy among counties in creating from scratch forms, processes, and procedures; and to forward an agenda of sustainability so that the initiative's success hinged not on individuals, but upon institutionalized structures in place. CCRWF also provided frequent technical assistance services to help counties develop and implement their coordinated approach at an accelerated pace.

Methods

Under an agreement with the Center for Social Services Research at the University of California at Berkeley (UCB), researchers conducted a process evaluation of the Linkages initiative. Telephone interviews were conducted in 2003, when many counties' efforts were relatively new, to establish a baseline understanding of goals, services, processes, successes, and barriers. In 2004, researchers conducted site visits, focus groups, and individual interviews with county staff to assess 10 programs considered by CCRWF and UCB to be in relatively mature states of implementation.

Each interview or focus group lasted approximately 1 1/2 hours. In four counties management and line staff were interviewed separately, and in four counties they were interviewed jointly, due to the small size of the group. The meeting schedule included managers but no line staff in one county, and line staff but no managers in another county. In some cases, the UCB team corresponded with managers after the interviews in order to clarify information that was not made clear during the site visits. Notes were handwritten during the interviews and later transcribed. The UCB evaluation team then used qualitative methods to analyze the data. The interview data were summarized for each county and then grouped according to themes that emerged.

A total of 104 individuals participated in the follow-up interviews. Of these participants, 26 were managers and 78 were line staff or supervisors in child welfare or CalWORKs. Interviewees varied in the length of time that they had worked in their respective county agencies. The mean duration of employment with an agency was 10 years, with a range of three months to 34 years.

A Coordinated Approach

There was significant variability across the counties in their approach to coordinated services. All counties conducted some type of coordinated case planning on behalf of dually-involved clients. In some cases child welfare and CalWORKs staff met to discuss the client's needs and resources; in other cases staff included parents in their meetings; and in still other counties joint staffing was used as an opportunity for multidisciplinary team meetings, including representatives from a range of agencies such as public health, mental health, substance abuse, and/or other service providers. Some counties used "linked case planning" to allow child welfare case plan requirements (e.g., parenting classes or substance abuse treatment) to "count" toward the welfare to work plan, or included welfare to work activities into the child welfare case plan. In the ideal model, goals, services, and timelines for child welfare and for welfare were coordinated.

Some counties used the Linkages initiative as an opportunity to co-locate services; in other counties, more traditional organizational structures remained, with communication encouraged through phone calls, meetings, and e-mail.

All counties attempted to target special populations either within the welfare caseload, or within child welfare. Rather than target families with known child or parental risk factors (such as those described previously), most agencies targeted Linkages services to TANF populations with known case characteristics (such as those soon-to-be sanctioned, or child-only cases).

In child welfare, most agency administrators targeted Linkages services to families at the front end of the system: either those recently reported to child welfare for maltreatment, or those receiving in-home services.

Challenges Along the Way

After four years of Linkages, the majority of counties had relatively strong programs operating either in pilot sites or county-wide. Although our work with counties did not allow us to assess outcomes for any of the families involved in Linkages, an assessment of the process of implementation suggests that efforts to coordinate services were not without their challenges. First among these was competition between diverse programmatic goals. County staff spent considerable time attempting to balance the need to promote self-sufficiency while at the same time supporting family stability. In principle, the goals were complementary, however, in practice there was sometimes friction: workers from TANF felt the need to push for family well-being through the avenue of work, while child welfare staff sometimes saw family well-being better facilitated through temporary non-work. Through regular communication between staff, most of these tensions dissipated over time, but they were exaggerated when staff experienced bureaucratic distance or had insufficient time to communicate with workers from the corresponding agency or unit.

Second, implementation was also slowed by an imbalance in organizational acceptance of the Linkages model. CalWORKs staff tended to be very enthusiastic about Linkages. Numerous CalWORKs interviewees reported increased job satisfaction, principally because they felt as though they were now making a substantive difference in their clients' lives. Workers were relieved to find ways *not* to sanction families, and this was frequently accomplished by allowing child welfare activities to count toward work hours. CalWORKs staff also were more familiar with the activities associated with coordinating services. Their history working with service providers in mental health, domestic violence, and substance abuse (mandated by California legislation) prior to the Linkages initiative gave them a degree of comfort with collaborative arrangements that was somewhat less customary for child welfare staff.

The enthusiasm exhibited by CalWORKs staff was contrasted by a general reluctance to embrace the new model of service delivery among child welfare workers. This, in spite of the fact that the benefits of Linkages appeared to be greatest for child welfare workers–in the form of sometimes reduced workloads and in terms of job satisfaction. And their clients often profited as well, particularly in the form of increased accessibility of services. Child welfare workers who used Linkages acknowledged that they had less antagonistic relationships with their clients due to the collaborative process, and that the sense of shared responsibility reduced job-related stress, but many child welfare staff were indisposed to participate largely because of perceived increases in workload.

The hesitancy in child welfare was not just organizational, but also philosophical. In many of the counties where we interviewed staff, child welfare workers were reluctant to acknowledge the place of poverty in their clients' lives, despite extensive research that demonstrates the connection between poverty and child maltreatment. Many staff became defensive about the suggestion that the majority of their clients are poor, and some cited examples of wealthy clients to contradict the link between poverty and maltreatment. Their hesitance may be psychologically protective against historical criticisms that child welfare workers remove children for reasons of poverty alone (Pelton, 1989), but it is paradoxical since the Linkages program was developed precisely because of the known intersect between these two compelling problems.

CONCLUSIONS

As other states and counties consider efforts to integrate welfare and child welfare services, they can benefit from the work that has gone before them in California and elsewhere (Berns & Drake, 1999; Ehrle,

Scarcella, & Geen, 2004). Further efforts to discern where, when, and with whom integrated services can and should be provided may differ from one locality to another, but some integrated services appear to be important in a reformed welfare environment. TANF reauthorization has been stalled in Washington D.C. for almost two years, but congressional discussions to date suggest that new iterations of reform are not likely to substantially change the tenor or approach of TANF policy. In fact, current proposals forwarded by the administration suggest a tightening of work requirements for low-income parents rather than an acknowledgement of the challenges posed by child-rearing in the context of poverty. A welfare policy landscape that is reliant on time limits and sanctions will likely increase material hardships for many families (Reichman, Teitler, & Curtis, 2005). As these parents struggle to raise their children, additional family support and social services may be necessary.

While the outcomes from an integrated services approach are as yet unclear, the knowledge base in the fields of welfare and child welfare is certainly substantial enough to consider targeting special services to those most likely to face difficulties parenting under conditions of poverty. Organizational and philosophical barriers may hamper the development of these efforts, but for families dually-involved in both welfare and child welfare systems, a coordinated approach holds promise for supporting child safety and family well-being.

REFERENCES

Berger, L.M., & Brooks-Gunn, J. (2005). Socioeconomic status, parenting knowledge and behaviors, and perceived maltreatment of young low-birth-weight children. *Social Service Review, 79*(2), 237-267.

Berns, D., & Drake, B.J. (March 1999). Combining child welfare and welfare reform at a local level. *Policy & Practice, 57*(1), 26-34.

Courtney, M., Piliavin, P., Dworsky, A., & Zinn, A. (2001). *Involvement of TANF Families with Child Welfare Services.* Paper presented at the Association of Public Policy Analysis and Management Research Meeting, Washington, DC, November 2, 2001.

Courtney, M., Piliavin, I., & Power, P. (2000). *Involvement of TANF Applicants with Child Protective Services.* Paper presented at the Association for Public Policy Analysis and Management Research Meeting, Seattle, Washington, November 2, 2000. URL: *http://www.ssc.wisc.edu/irp/*

Derr, M., & Taylor, M. (2004). The link between childhood and adult abuse among long-term welfare recipients. *Children and Youth Services Review, 26*(2), 173-184.

Ehrle, J., Scarcella, C., & Geen, R. (2004). Teaming up: Collaboration between welfare and child welfare agencies since welfare reform. *Children and Youth Services Review, 26*(3), 265-285.

Fein, D., & Lee, W. (2003). The impacts of welfare reform on child maltreatment in Delaware. *Children and Youth Services Review, 25*(1), 83-111.

Frame, L. (1999). Suitable homes revisited: An historical look at child protection and welfare reform. *Children and Youth Services Review, 21*(9/10), 719-754.

Frame, L., & Berrick, J.D. (2003). The effects of welfare reform on families involved with public child welfare services: Results from a qualitative study. *Children and Youth Services Review, 25*(1-2), 113-138.

Geen, R., Fender, L., Leos-Urbel, J., & Markowitz, T. (2001). *Welfare Reform's Effects on Child Welfare Caseloads.* Washington, DC: Urban Institute.

Geen, R., & Tumlin, K. (1999). *State Efforts to Remake Child Welfare: Responses to New Challenges and Increased Scrutiny.* Washington, DC: Urban Institute.

Ginsberg, L.H. (2001). *Careers in Social Work.* Boston, MA: Allyn & Bacon.

Needell, B., Cuccaro-Alamin, S., Brookhart, A., & Lee, S. (1999). Transitions from AFDC to child welfare in California. *Children and Youth Services Review, 21*(9-10), 815-841.

Nightingale, D.S., Kramer, F.D., Trutko, J., Egner, M., & Barnow, B. (2003). *The Role of One-Stop Career Centers in Serving Welfare Recipients in 2002.* Prepared for the U.S. Department of Labor, Employment and Training Annual Research Conference, Washington, DC.

Ovwhigo, P., Leavitt, K., & Born, C. (2003). Risk factors for child abuse and neglect among former TANF families: Do later leavers experience greater risk? *Children and Youth Services Review, 25*(1-2), 139-163.

Paxson, C., & Waldfogel, J. (1999). *Work, Welfare, and Child Maltreatment.* Working Paper 7343. National Bureau of Economic Research. Cambridge, MA. URL: *http://www.nber.org/papers/w7343.*

Paxson, C., & Waldfogel, J. (2001). Welfare reforms, family resources, and child maltreatment. In B. Meyer & G. Duncan (Eds.), *The Incentives of Government Programs and the Well-Being of Families,* pp. 1-47. Chicago: Joint Center for Poverty Research.

Pelton, L.H. (1989). *For Reasons of Poverty: A Critical Analysis of the Public Child Welfare System in the United States.* New York: Praeger.

Reichman, N.E., Teitler, J.O., & Curtis, M.A. (2005). TANF sanctioning and hardship. *Social Service Review, 79*(2): 215-236.

Sedlak, A.J., & Broadhurst, D.D. (1996). *Third National Incidence Study of Child Abuse and Neglect: Final Report.* Washington, DC: U.S. Department of Health and Human Services, Administration for Children and Families, Administration on Children, Youth and Families, National Center on Child Abuse and Neglect.

Shook, K. (1999). Does the loss of welfare income increase the risk of involvement with the child welfare system? *Children and Youth Services Review, 21*(9-10), 781-814.

Slack, K., Holl, J., Lee, B., McDaniel, M., Altenbernd, L., & Stevens, A. (2003). Child protective intervention in the context of welfare reform: The effects of work and welfare on maltreatment reports. *Journal of Policy Analysis and Management,* *22*(4), 517-536.

Thompson, T.S., Van Nexx, A., & O'Brien, C.T. (2001). *Screening and Assessment in TANF/Welfare to Work: Local Answers to Difficult Questions.* Administration for Children and Families & Office of the Assistant Secretary for Planning and Evaluation. U.S. Department of Health and Human Services.

U.S. Department of Health and Human Services, Administration on Children, Youth and Families (2003). *Child Maltreatment 2003.* Washington, DC: U.S. Government Printing Office, 2005c. Retrieved June 22, 2005 from the World Wide Web: *http://www.acf.hhs.gov/programs/cb/publications/cmreports.htm*

U.S. Department of Health and Human Services (2002). *Child Maltreatment 2002.* Washington, DC: Children's Bureau.

U.S. House of Representatives, Committee on Ways and Means (2004). *2004 Green Book.* Washington, DC: U.S. Government Printing Office.

Waldfogel, J. (2004). Welfare reform and the child welfare system. *Children and Youth Services Review, 26*(10): 919-939.

Wells, K.,& Guo, S. (2003). Mothers' welfare and work, income and reunification with children in foster care. *Children and Youth Services Review, 25*(3): 203-224.

Wells, K., & Guo, S. (2004). Reunification of foster children before and after welfare reform. *Social Services Review, 78*(1): 76-95.

A Rose by Any Other Name?
Lump-Sum Diversion
or Traditional Welfare Grant?

Andrea Hetling
Kirk Tracy
Catherine E. Born

SUMMARY. Critics of diversion grants, lump-sum payments designed to alleviate short-term emergencies and prevent the need for ongoing Temporary Assistance to Needy Families (TANF) receipt, claim that recipients use monetary amounts similar to traditional welfare recipients. This paper examines the total cash grants for two cohorts of TANF applicants: those whose applications resulted in a TANF grant and those who received a diversion grant. Multivariate regression models show that diversion leads to a reduction of $1,841.44 in cash benefit receipt during

Andrea Hetling, PhD, is affiliated with the Department of Public Policy, University of Connecticut. Kirk Tracy, PhD, and Catherine E. Born, PhD, are affiliated with the School of Social Work, University of Maryland.

Address correspondence to: Andrea Hetling, PhD, Assistant Professor, Department of Public Policy, University of Connecticut, 1800 Asylum Avenue, West Hartford, CT 06117 (E-mail: andrea.hetling@uconn.edu).

A portion of these findings was presented at the 26th Annual Association for Policy Analysis and Management Conference on October 29, 2004.

The research was supported by funding from the Maryland Department of Human Resources.

[Haworth co-indexing entry note]: "A Rose by Any Other Name? Lump Sum Diversion or Traditional Welfare Grant?" Hetling, Andrea, Kirk Tracy, and Catherine E. Born. Co-published simultaneously in *Journal of Policy Practice* (The Haworth Press, Inc.) Vol. 5, No. 2/3, 2006, pp. 43-59; and: *International Perspectives on Welfare to Work Policy* (ed: Richard Hoefer, and James Midgley) The Haworth Press, Inc., 2006, pp. 43-59. Single or multiple copies of this article are available for a fee from The Haworth Document Delivery Service [1-800-HAWORTH, 9:00 a.m. - 5:00 p.m. (EST). E-mail address: docdelivery@haworthpress.com].

the three-year tracking period (p < 0.001). Findings suggest that diversion payments are not TANF under another name. *[Article copies available for a fee from The Haworth Document Delivery Service: 1-800-HAWORTH. E-mail address: <docdelivery@haworthpress.com> Website: <http://www.HaworthPress. com> © 2006 by The Haworth Press, Inc. All rights reserved.]*

KEYWORDS. Welfare, diversion, Temporary Assistance to Needy Families (TANF)

INTRODUCTION

Diversion strategies, established by the 1996 federal welfare reform legislation, the Personal Responsibility and Work Opportunities Reconciliation Act (PRWORA), are alleged to be innovative techniques to help families avoid welfare dependency. The premise of diversion is that monthly cash grants may not be the best way of helping poor families in all cases and other, more appropriate, services may enable them to become self-sufficient without ever entering the "rolls." In many states, including Maryland, diversion allows potential Temporary Assistance to Needy Families (TANF) recipients to collect one large lump-sum payment, so that rather than receiving smaller monthly TANF checks, individuals receive the equivalent of several months of benefits at once in order to alleviate an immediate crisis, such as an urgent automobile repair or avoiding an eviction. The only restriction is that they are then ineligible to receive TANF for the equivalent number of months.

Diversion grants are especially appealing in these times of budget shortfalls as it is assumed that one-time lump-sum grants are less costly than traditional, longer-term, cash assistance. This assumption, however, has not been unequivocally determined. Some scholars believe that diversion strategies are as costly as monthly grants and, moreover, do not offer the same incentives such as time limits and work requirements as TANF does (Besharov & Germanis, 2004). Also, if work participation rates increase with TANF reauthorization, diversion could be used as a way for states to reduce the number of people required to work and thus increase their rates through legerdemain.

This study examines a critical assumption about the nature of diversion programs. That is, are diversion programs, specifically lump-sum cash grants, a cost effective alternative to traditional monthly cash grant programs? Are diverted clients actually "diverted" from welfare or are they just using equivalent funds in a different way?

Using Maryland State administrative data, this study compares the total receipt of cash grants over a three-year period of two welfare applicant cohorts, those whose application resulted in a Welfare Avoidance Grant (WAG) and those who became new TANF clients. The cohort of individuals who received a WAG between October 1, 1999 and December 31, 1999 (n = 315) was matched on two criteria, region and number of adults, to a sample of new TANF recipients of the same time period. Data on the two groups' use of cash grants, both WAGs and TANF, over 36 months were tracked and calculated. Additionally, an Ordinary Least Squares regression model was designed with other demographic and life experience controls to determine whether or not WAG receipt resulted in a lesser amount of cash assistance during the 36-month outcome period. The findings are important not only for Maryland, but also for other states implementing and developing policies related to diversion grants. Many states have lump-sum programs similar to Maryland's; others may also be able to design similar studies specifically for their own state's program.

BACKGROUND

While a few studies have examined the prevalence and characteristics of diverted clients (for a review, see Lacey, Hetling, & Born, 2002; London, 2003), little research has been done to determine whether diversion strategies actually divert or merely delay cash assistance or whether diversion programs are a cost-effective alternative to monthly cash assistance receipt. Research on diversion is lacking partly because such strategies were not a part of pre-reform state waiver experiments. Moreover, as per the design of TANF, states have great leeway in their use of diversion programs, if they choose to implement diversion programs at all. The three forms of formal diversion programs, lump-sum payments, job search, and alternative resources, can be offered independently or in any combination (for more information, see Lacey, Hetling, & Born, 2002). This flexibility, while programmatically beneficial, poses great barriers for evaluation and research on diversion programs. Additionally, some research has highlighted the use of informal diversion tactics, or techniques or methods that hinder or deter an individual's successful completion of the application process.

This study focuses on formal diversion strategies and, in particular, lump-sum payments, the most widely used of the three formal types of diversion. As of this writing, 30 states currently offer some sort of cash diversion program (Administration for Children & Families, 2002). Among the states that offer lump-sum payment programs, there are also variations in the amount of money an individual is allowed to receive at one given time and five states allow counties to determine how they want to implement their programs (Administration for Children & Families, 2002).

The lack of program data on diverted clients and their families poses another research obstacle. Because certain types of diverted clients are never formally enrolled in TANF, they are not usually tracked in administrative data systems (London, 2003). Even when the diversion event has been documented in the state's system, the data required for programmatic purposes are often not detailed enough for research purposes and do not provide a clear picture of the circumstances surrounding the diversion event or the characteristics of the family.

As a result of these barriers to research on diversion, most research efforts are state-specific, resulting in a handful of state-level reports and only one national study to date. The national study utilized the 1999 National Survey of America's Families (NSAF), and focused on recipients of lump-sum payments (London, 2003). The study analyzed the characteristics of diverted clients and found that diversion programs may be targeting two distinct groups: job-ready applicants with high levels of education and unprepared applicants with low education levels who perhaps opt for the larger sum of money and attempt to save future months of TANF. The study also analyzed the outcomes of diverted clients in comparison to TANF leavers in terms of employment outcomes and Food Stamps and Medicaid receipt.

The interpretation of the findings of this national study is more cautious in attributing success to diversion programs than are most of the state-level studies that have been conducted up to this point. To date, there have been a number of state studies conducted on diversion programs (Assistant Secretary for Planning and Evaluation, 2002). State-level outcome studies have focused on recidivism rates of diverted clients and have found that diverted clients returned to cash assistance at slightly less or comparable rates as TANF leavers (Goldsmith & Valvano, 2002; Lacey et al., 2002; Schexnayder, Schroeder, Lein, Dominguez, Douglas, & Richards, 2002).

Of the studies that have looked at the potential savings of diversion, the initial results seem positive. A study on South Dakota's diversion program concluded that one $300 payment, the average monthly benefit for the typical South Dakota AFDC recipient, can save taxpayers nearly $7,000 (U.S. Department of Labor, Employment & Training Administration, 2003). Thus, it has been alleged that the $40,000 spent on diversion payments for 134 potential welfare applicants theoretically saved South Dakota more than $900,000 in roughly two years (U.S. Department of Labor, Employment & Training Administration, 2003). A study on Colorado's diversion program has estimated that the State saves as much as $5.4 million annually by helping people avoid spells on TANF through its program (Goldsmith & Valvano, 2002). Furthermore, a comparison of Kentucky's diversion program and cash assistance program has shown that Kentucky saves $347 a year per diversion case, producing an annual savings of over $2 million (Barber, Daugherty, & McAdams, 2002).

The research presented here addresses this issue of cost by calculating the amount of cash grants for two cohorts of TANF applicants: those whose applications resulted in the award of a "regular" TANF grant and those whose applications resulted in issuance of a WAG. The major question guiding our research is: Do diverted clients receive more or less cash through the WAGs and subsequent monthly cash assistance (if applicable) than do individuals receiving monthly TANF grants? While our question is not new, the methods used distinguish our research from previous studies and add to the current literature in two important ways. First, the study utilizes a longer follow-up period than other state studies. Second, we control for differences in background characteristics through the use of matching samples and regression techniques, a critical method considering the large, identified differences between diverters and TANF recipients.

METHODS

Samples

Between October 1, 1999 and December 31, 1999 a total of 5,372 individuals applied for TANF and subsequently were issued either a WAG (n = 325) or began a TANF spell (n = 5,047). Chi-square and ANOVA tests were conducted between the two cohorts on the variables of race, region, number of adults, number of children, and marital status. Based on theory and the bivariate data analyses, the variables of region and number of adults were chosen as the matching criteria for the cohorts.

Differences between the cohorts in terms of region stood out as being both statistically significant and very large. Moreover, in other research, region, in particular urban versus suburban or rural differences, has consistently been noted as an important determinant in welfare exit and dependency (for example, Allen & Kirby, 2000). In order to ensure that outcome differences between the two groups could not be attributed solely to this variable, recipients within the two groups were separated into their respective regions.

Chi-square and ANOVA tests were subsequently performed on the variables of race, number of adults, number of children, and marital status for the regional groups. During these analyses, statistically significant differences in the number of adults per case were consistently found between the two groups, in all regions. Again, the number of adults is often included in analyses as a predictor of welfare dependency or self-sufficiency; two-parent cases fare differently than one-parent assistance units and differently again from "child-only" cases where the adult on the case is not eligible for benefits (Wood & Strong, 2002). In order to ensure that outcome differences between the groups could not be attributed to this factor, the variable measuring number of adults was also used as a matching criterion.

Using these two dimensions, the study sample was then narrowed down to two groups. Each group was matched on region and the number of adults, and consisted of 315 persons. In each matched pair, one sample member received a WAG in October, November, or December of 1999, and the other began a new TANF spell during the same time period. Table 1, below, shows the number and percentage of recipients from each region and the breakdown for the number of adults on each case.

TABLE 1. Matching Variable Frequencies

Matching Criteria	WAG recipients	TANF recipients
Region		
Baltimore City	2 (0.6%)	2 (0.6%)
Prince George's County	5 (1.6%)	5 (1.6%)
Metro Region	131 (41.6%)	131 (41.6%)
Southern Maryland	79 (25.1%)	79 (25.1%)
Western Maryland	33 (10.5%)	33 (10.5%)
Upper Shore	9 (2.9%)	9 (2.9%)
Lower Shore	56 (17.8%)	56 (17.8%)
Number of Adults		
0	2 (0.6%)	2 (0.6%)
1	275 (87.3%)	275 (87.3%)
2	38 (12.1%)	38 (12.1%)

Notes: The Metro Region is made up of Baltimore, Montgomery, Carroll, Harford, Howard, and Frederick Counties. Southern Maryland included Anne Arundel, Calvert, Charles, and St. Mary's Counties. Western Maryland consisted of Garrett, Allegany, and Washington Counties. The Upper Shore consisted of Cecil, Kent, Queen Anne's, Caroline, Talbot, and Dorchester Counties, and the Lower Shore consisted of Worcester, Wicomico, and Somerset Counties.

Data Sources

Findings for this report were based on data retrieved by the authors from three different Maryland state administrative data systems. All demographic characteristics and program participation data were obtained from the Automated Information Management System/Automated Master File (AIMS/AMF) and the Client Automated Resources and Eligibility System (CARES). CARES is the official statewide automated data system for public welfare programs overseen by the Department of Human Resources and includes information on individual and case level program participation data for cash assistance, Food Stamps, Medical Assistance and Social Services, as well as important demographic information. AIMS/AMF was the predecessor to CARES, which officially replaced AIMS/AMF in 1998. Although no new data have been entered into AIMS/AMF since 1998, it is still a valuable resource for data regarding historical program participation.

Information regarding employment and earnings was obtained via the Maryland Automated Benefits System (MABS), which contains data on all Unemployment Insurance-covered jobs in Maryland. Examples of jobs not tracked within this system include federal government employees (civilian and military), independent contractors, commission-only salespersons, most religious organization employees, some student interns, self-employed persons with no paid staff, and farm workers. "Under the table" jobs are not included, nor are ones that are located outside of Maryland.

Analyses

Data from the above sources were used to profile demographic characteristics, welfare and employment experiences of the two cohorts. This profile is intended to provide a description of the groups and aid in understanding background differences between the groups both for programmatic and statistical purposes. Bivariate analyses, specifically Chi-square and ANOVA tests, were used to examine the differences.

Multivariate analyses were used to examine the primary outcome measure, total cash benefit receipt, during the three-year tracking period of the two cohorts, controlling for a number of background characteristics, and were based on the following model.

$$\text{Outcome} = \alpha + \beta_{\text{WAG}} + \beta X_{\text{Demographics}} + \beta X_{\text{Work/welfare history}} + \beta_{\text{City residence}} + \varepsilon$$

The WAG variable measures the impact of WAG receipt on the outcome variable. Because the TANF recipient cohort served as the control or reference group, TANF receipt was not included in the model. The matrices of demographic and work and welfare history variables were included in the model as important independent variables that likely influence the outcome variable. Demographic variables included age in years at the critical study date, sex (female = 1, male = 0), race (African American = 1, other = 0), marital status (never married = 1, other = 0), number of children, and number of adults (one adult cases were the reference group with child-only and more than one adult variables in the model). Work and welfare historical variables included the number of quarters employed over the past eight calendar quarters or two years, employment status at the critical study date, earnings in $1,000s in quarter of critical study date, and number of months of TANF receipt out of the past 60 months. Lastly, City residence was included in the model as an independent variable.

As previously explained, the outcome or dependent variable covered a three-year follow-up period. The follow-up period began with the receipt of a check (WAG or regular) and the dependent variable was total cash benefit receipt. This continuous variable measures the total amount of cash received through either TANF or WAG checks during the three-year follow-up period. The average receipt for the sample members was $3,247 with a standard deviation of $3,093. The range of cash received was between $117 and $17,636. Although the cohorts were matched on two critical variables, differences in other background characteristics merited the use of multivariate analyses to ensure that any observed outcome differences were not attributable to baseline differences such as employment status or historical welfare receipt. In short, we ask the following: holding individual background characteristics constant, do WAG recipients receive more or less cash assistance than TANF recipients? Ordinary Least Squares (OLS) regression was used to analyze the model. This type of multivariate regression model is used when the dependent variable is of a continuous nature. The raw coefficients are interpreted as a one-unit change in the independent variable leads to an x unit change in the outcome or dependent variable.

BASELINE CHARACTERISTICS

While we were not able to match the two groups on all background characteristics, the demographic profiles are very similar. Out of the seven demographic variables not used in the matching process, very small, but statistically significant differences were found on three measures. Moreover, WAG and TANF recipients were found to be statistically equal on the remaining four measures, as highlighted in Table 2. Table 2 also presents data on the historical employment experiences and usage of Temporary Cash Assistance (TANF), Food Stamps, and Medical Assistance for the two cohorts.

TABLE 2. Baseline Characteristics of WAG Recipients vs. TANF Recipients

Characteristics	WAG Recipients (n = 315)	TANF Recipients (n = 315)	Entire Sample (n = 630)
Payee's Gender			
Female (n)	95.9% (302)	94.6% (298)	95.2% (600)
Payee's Age*			
Mean (Standard Deviation)	31.38 (7.81)	29.98 (8.52)	30.68 (8.20)
Range	18 to 55	18 to 65	18 to 65
Payee's Age at First Birth			
Mean (Standard Deviation)	22.13 (5.24)	21.39 (5.12)	21.78 (5.19)
Range	14 to 42	11 to 41	11 to 42
Payee's Racial/Ethnic Background			
African American (n)	53.0% (160)	53.8% (164)	53.4% (324)
Caucasian (n)	45.4% (137)	43.6% (133)	44.5% (270)
Other (n)	1.7% (5)	2.6% (8)	2.1% (13)
Marital Status*			
Never Married (n)	49.2% (155)	61.6% (194)	55.4% (349)
Number of Children**			
Mean (Standard Deviation)	2.04 (1.17)	1.77 (1.24)	1.91 (1.21)
Range	0 to 8	0 to 9	0 to 9
Age of Youngest Child			
Mean (Standard Deviation)	5.54 (4.49)	5.24 (4.79)	5.39 (4.64)
Range	< 1 mo to 17 yrs	< 1 mo to 18 years	< 1 mo to 18 yrs
Households with a child under 3 (n)	37.1% (115)	43.4% (126)	40.2% (241)
UI-Covered Employment			
8 Quarters before study date			
Percent Working***	93.0%	80.6%	86.8%
Mean Quarters Worked***	5.46	3.84	4.65
Mean Quarterly Earnings***	$2,588	$1,544	$2,066
Quarter of study date			
Percent Working***	79.4%	43.8%	61.6%
Mean Earnings***	$2,287	$589	$1,438
Months of TANF Receipt in			
Previous 5 Years*			
Mean (Standard Deviation)	12.13 (14.50)	14.90 (16.61)	13.51 (15.64)
Previous Year			
Mean (Standard Deviation)	1.01 (2.31)	1.25 (2.46)	1.13 (2.39)

Notes: *p < .05 **p < .01 ***p < .001

Although statistically significant differences were found for three demographic measures, the practical differences between the values were actually quite small. WAG recipients were, on average, slightly older than TANF recipients, with a mean age of 31.38 years compared to 29.98 years. Slightly less than half (49.2%) of WAG recipients had never been married, compared to approximately three out of five (61.6%) TANF recipients. A final area of difference between the two cohorts was in the average number of children per household. The typical WAG household contained 2.04 children, while the typical TANF household had 1.77 children.

In comparing patterns of employment before and during the critical study quarter, WAG recipients were more likely to have worked and earned more than TANF recipients and the difference between the two cohorts was statistically significant on each measure analyzed. In the eight quarters, or two years, preceding the critical study date, more than nine of every 10 (93.0%) WAG recipients worked at some point, averaging a total of 5.46 quarters during that period. In comparison, slightly more than eight of every 10 (80.6%) TANF recipients worked at all during the same period and the average time spent employed was 3.84 quarters. During this period WAG recipients earned on average $16,875, almost double the amount earned by TANF recipients ($8,747). The differences in employment were greatest between the two cohorts in the last quarter of 1999, the calendar quarter containing the critical study date. During that quarter almost eight of 10 (79.4%) WAG recipients worked while less than half (43.8%) of TANF recipients were employed. The typical WAG recipient earned an average of $2,287, nearly four times the average ($589) earned by TANF recipients.

In general, even statistically significant differences between the two groups in the measures of welfare use were quite small. Regarding TANF receipt in the prior year, WAG recipients received an average of 1.01 months of assistance, compared to 1.25 months for TANF recipients. While statistically significant, the difference in TANF receipt in the five years preceding the critical study date was less than three months with WAG recipients averaging 12.13 months of TANF receipt and TANF recipients averaging 14.90 months.

RECEIPT OF CASH GRANTS OVER THREE YEARS

Table 3 presents information comparing the cash benefits (WAG and TANF) received by the two cohorts in the three-year period beginning with the benefit that brought them into our sample. Table 4 contains the results of an Ordinary Least Squares regression analysis examining the amount of cash assistance received in the 36-month follow-up period controlling for a number of background characteristics. Table 3 is divided into three sections in order to describe the differences in the type of cash assistance received by the two groups. Table 4 focuses only on the total amount of cash, regardless of the type of assistance. All of the differences mentioned in the following discussion are statistically significant.

Descriptive Findings

As seen in Table 3, WAG recipients averaged fewer TANF benefit checks (1.83) than TANF recipients (11.68). The more than five-to-one

TABLE 3. Total Receipt of Cash Grants During 36-Month Tracking Period

	WAG Recipients (n = 315)	TANF Recipients (n = 315)	Entire Sample (n = 630)
TANF receipt			
Number of Checks***			
Mean (Standard Deviation)	1.83 (4.44)	11.68 (8.52)	6.76 (8.39)
Median	0.00	9.00	4.00
Range	0 to 33	1 to 37	0 to 37
Total Amount***			
Mean	$640	$4,140	$2,390
Median	$0.00	$3,026	$1,228
Standard Deviation	$1,601	$3,562	$3,268
Range	$0 to $11,032	$207 to $17,636	$0 to $17,636
WAG Receipt			
Number of Checks***			
Mean (Standard Deviation)	1.36 (0.82)	0.06 (0.32)	0.71 (0.90)
Median	1.00	0.00	1.00
Range	1 to 8	0 to 4	0 to 8
Total Amount***			
Mean (Standard Deviation)	$1,634 ($1,443)	$79 ($434)	$857 ($1,319)
Median	$1,212	$0.00	$318
Range	$117 to $9,011	$0 to $4,152	$0 to $9,011
All Cash Assistance (TANF and WAG)			
Number of Checks***			
Mean (Standard Deviation)	3.19 (4.50)	11.74 (8.49)	7.46 (8.01)
Median	1.00	9.00	5.00
Range	1 to 34	1 to 37	1 to 37
Total Amount***			
Mean (Standard Deviation)	$2,274 ($2,161)	$4,219 ($3,549)	$3,247 ($3,093)
Median	$1,500	$3,106	$2,254
Range	$117 to $12,622	$207 to $17,636	$117 to $17,636

Notes: *p < .05 **p < .01 ***p < .001

ratio in checks received translated to a similar proportion of TANF monies received, as WAG recipients averaged $640, compared to $4,140 received by TANF recipients. In contrast, during the three-year tracking period, WAG recipients received a greater number of WAG checks (1.36) on average than did TANF recipients (0.06 TANF checks). On average, WAG recipients also received a much larger sum of money in WAGs than did members of the TANF cohort ($1,634 vs. $79, respectively).

TABLE 4. Ordinary Least Squares Regression Predicting Cash Benefit Receipt

Predictor	Model (1)	Model (2)	Model (3)	Model (4)
WAG recipient	−1944.957*** (234.127)	−2081.515*** (232.174)	−1812.203*** (261.081)	−1841.438*** (258.335)
Age		1.362 (15.212)	−3.676 (15.570)	−0.970 (15.416)
Sex		408.449 (555.701)	366.358 (558.726)	368.315 (552.611)
Race		−18.094 (247.003)	4.729 (253.828)	−58.745 (251.595)
Marital Status		256.273 (254.411)	243.212 (254.999)	285.405 (252.448)
Number of children		590.260*** (99.261)	565.160*** (99.772)	558.179*** (98.696)
Child-only case		166.025 (1670.352)	493.048 (1675.789)	470.887 (1657.458)
More than 1 adult on case		145.067 (367.494)	207.359 (374.568)	231.090 (370.520)
Employment history			−30.785 (45.426)	−24.746 (44.957)
Employment status at critical study date			−511.897 (292.019)	−499.836 (288.840)
Earnings in $1000s in quarter of critical study date			0.008 (0.065)	0.014 (0.065)
TANF history			13.143 (7.951)	10.994 (7.883)
City residence				5489.201*** (1431.265)
R^2	0.099	0.153	0.164	0.183
Sample Size	630	630	630	630

Notes: $*p < 0.05$, $**p < 0.01$, $***p < 0.001$

Overall, examining both forms of assistance, WAG recipients received fewer benefit checks for less total cash than did TANF recipients. WAG cohort members received an average of 3.19 checks in comparison to the average of 11.74 checks received by TANF cohort members. More importantly, the total cash utilized by WAG recipients ($2,274) was approximately half of what was received by TANF customers ($4,219).

Multivariate Findings

Table 4 presents findings from an Ordinary Least Squares regression analysis examining cash benefit receipt as a function of WAG receipt and other background characteristics. Although the initial intent of creating two matched cohorts was to eliminate differences in baseline characteristics, the statistical tests conducted between the groups showed that a few important differences remained. Thus, in order to control for these differences, a series of models were designed with each successive model including additional variables to determine which act as predictors for future cash benefit receipt.

The first model examines the correlation between our policy variable of interest, WAG receipt, and total cash benefit receipt in the follow-up period. A statistically significant, negative relationship was found between WAG receipt and cash benefit receipt. Specifically, according to Model (1), without accounting for any other variables, the receipt of a WAG, as opposed to TANF, led to a $1,944.96 decrease in the follow-up cash total received.

In addition to measuring the effects of WAG receipt, Model 2 also looked at age, sex, race, marital status, number of children, child only cases, and having more than one adult on a case. Once again, even when controlling for the other variables, a negative significant relationship was found to exist between WAG receipt and cash benefit receipt at the $p < 0.001$ level. Model 2 found that those who received a WAG received $2,081.51 less than TANF recipients. The only other variable found to be significantly correlated with cash benefit receipt in this model was number of children, also at the $p < 0.001$ level, but this was a positive relationship. As the number of children increased, so did cash benefit receipt by $590.26.

In addition to the aforementioned variables, Model (3) includes employment history over the past two years, employment status in the critical study quarter, earnings in $1,000s in quarter of the critical study date, and historical months of TANF during the previous five years. Surprisingly, none of the newly added variables were statistically significant although differences between the two cohorts on these measures were notable in the bivariate analyses. The number of children continued to be statistically correlated with total cash benefits as did WAG receipt. Receiving a WAG reduced cash benefit receipt by $1,812.20 during the 36-month period, and each additional child on the grant increased cash benefit receipt by $565.16.

Model (4), the final model, added city residence as a factor in cash benefit receipt to the previously mentioned variables. In this model, both city residence and number of children were found to have positive significant relationships with cash benefit receipt. Living in the city increased cash benefit receipt by $5,489.20, while each additional child increased cash benefit receipt by $558.18. When controlling for all other variables, Model (4) shows that the impact of WAG receipt remains robust, leading to a reduction of $1,841.44 in total cash benefit receipt during the three-year tracking period. This relationship remains statistically significant at the $p < 0.001$ level.

DISCUSSION AND CONCLUSION

Welfare Avoidance Grants were designed to help those families who, under normal circumstances, are most likely able to be self-sufficient, but due to extenuating circumstances find themselves temporarily unable to make ends meet or are in a position where without some immediate financial help will soon be unable to do so. Briefly stated, recipients of WAGs, according to these data, are making minimal use of cash benefits in comparison to new TANF recipients. On average, WAG recipients received one-fourth the number of total assistance checks during the three-year tracking period and approximately half the amount of cash that TANF recipients did ($2,274 vs. $4,219, respectively). After controlling for a number of baseline characteristics using multivariate regression analyses, the receipt of a WAG as opposed to TANF led to a $1,841.44 reduction in the amount of cash benefits received during the three-year tracking period.

Although these numbers may suggest that WAG program participants have better outcomes than those receiving TANF and that perhaps the WAG program is more "successful" or "effective" than TANF, this type of inference is not valid. Although WAG customers do need to qualify for TANF before receiving a WAG, financial eligibility is not the only criterion used to determine whether or not someone receives a WAG. WAG recipients are supposed to be, by definition, those who have a high likelihood of being able to remain independent after receiving a WAG, obviously a factor not taken into consideration before someone is granted TANF. Moreover, although differences in employment experiences were not statistically significant in the multivariate models, a variety of unobservable or unmeasured characteristics may be at play. For example, WAG recipients may have negative attitudes towards traditional monthly assistance or may have jobs in better industries than do TANF recipients. Both factors would logically influence the receipt of cash benefits in the tracking period. Alternatively, perhaps WAG recipients have the perception that it is too difficult to qualify for monthly aid and are thus deterred from submitting another application. Because of these unanswered questions, it is impossible to attribute the identified impact to the policy alone and not partially to the attributes of the participants.

Even after taking these considerations into account, however, the results of this study seem to suggest that the WAG program is fulfilling its implied promise of helping at-risk families without entangling them in a long-term (or costly) relationship with public assistance. With a large proportion of WAG recipients able to make minimal use of initial cash grants and forego additional assistance, these data indicate that caseworkers are correctly identifying those who would benefit most from a WAG. Additionally, findings indicate that once those people have been correctly identified, the program has been sufficient in helping them remain off of assistance. Although results indicate that individuals who receive WAGs have benefited from the program, our findings cannot determine whether or not caseworkers are under-identifying individuals. It is possible, especially considering how relatively few individuals had participated in the program, at least during the later months of 1999, that other potential recipients who have not been offered a WAG or have turned it down because they do not fully understand this new program may also succeed with the help of a WAG. At the other extreme, we would caution that most likely WAGs are not appropriate strategies for all TANF applicants and should not be universally granted.

We conclude that recipients of lump-sum diversion payments do use less cash assistance than TANF recipients and that, at least in our study state, diversion is not simply TANF under a different name. The program appears to be one positive innovation resulting from the 1996 welfare reform legislation, and is further evidence of the need for innovative thinking when struggling with the challenges inherent in running a social service program within the confines of a budget. The objectives of assisting families and reducing the welfare rolls may seem paradoxical in nature. However, innovative programs such as lump-sum payments illustrate that it is possible to provide relief to those in need while at the same time reducing costs and providing financial aid to families without enmeshing them in "welfare."

Regardless of the preliminary nature of the findings and a degree of uncertainty due to possible selection bias, we feel sufficiently confident in the findings and continued potential of diversion to present two groups of recommendations. First, agency policy and frontline practice should continue to make use of diversion strategies, with a degree of caution, for those clients struggling with short-term crises. In addition, it would benefit future research endeavors as well as the clients themselves to interview those diverted clients who return to the rolls regarding the reasons for their return and the perceived benefit provided by the lump-sum payment program.

Second, as with so many other research projects, the answers to these research questions have led to other important ones. Specifically, questions regarding background differences and identifying potential recipients are very important and merit further attention perhaps with research focused on subgroup analyses. Diversion strategies were designed for and are targeted to individuals experiencing specific situations. Identified background differences in age, race, marital status, place of residence, and child-only cases beg the question of how participation in diversion programs as opposed to TANF affects different groups. While the effect of a WAG seems positive for the general group of recipients, perhaps future research will be able to identify certain subgroups who benefit more or less from this strategy. This is particularly important given criticisms that the use of diversion strategies may increase dramatically if states choose to use lump-sum grants as a way to meet stricter work participation rates.

REFERENCES

Administration for Children & Families (2002). *Applicant cash diversion programs.* Washington, DC: Author. Retrieved May, 14, 2003 from *http://www.acf.hhs.gov/ programs/ofa/annualreport5*

Allen, K., & Kirby, M. (2000). *Unfinished business: Why cities matter to welfare reform.* The Brookings Institution Survey Series. Washington, DC: The Brookings Institution.

Barber, G., Daugherty, B., & McAdams, D. (August, 2002). *An alternative to TANF: Experience with Kentucky's Family Alternative Diversion Program.* Conference paper presented at NAWRS 42nd Annual Workshop.

Besharov, B., & Germanis, P. (2004). *Toughening TANF: How much? And how attainable?* Washington, DC: American Enterprise Institute.

Goldsmith, D., & Valvano, V. (August, 2002). *TANF diversion: An effective strategy for helping families remain off assistance?* Conference paper presented at: NAWRS 42nd Annual Workshop.

Lacey, D., Hetling, A., & Born, C.E. (2002). *Life without welfare: The prevalence and outcomes of diversion strategies in Maryland.* Baltimore, MD: University of Maryland School of Social Work.

London, R.A. (2003). Which TANF applicants are diverted, and what are their outcomes. *Social Service Review,* 77(3):373-398.

Loprest, P.J. (2003). Use of government benefits increases among families leaving welfare. *Snapshots of America's families III,* No. 6. Washington, DC: The Urban Institute.

Schexnayder, D., Schroeder, D., Lein, L., Dominguez, D., Douglas, K., & Richards, F. (2002). *Surviving Without TANF: An analysis of families diverted from or leaving TANF.* Austin, TX: Texas Department of Human Services.

U.S. Department of Labor, Employment & Training Administration. *Welfare diversion project: State of South Dakota program highlights.* Retrieved November 10, 2003 from *http://wtw.doleta.gov/documents/casebook/allcasewd.asp*

Wood, R., & Strong, D. (2002). *The status of families on child-only TANF cases.* Princeton, NJ: Mathematica Policy Research, Inc.

Welfare to Work
in the United Kingdom

Martin Evans
Jane Millar

SUMMARY. Increasing employment and reducing child poverty are two central goals of current government welfare reform policy in the UK, and single parents–with their relatively low employment rates and relatively high poverty rates–are one of the key target groups for both. This article outlines welfare reform policies in the UK with particular reference to single parents, and discusses the impact of these. In doing so, it highlights some key differences compared with the US. *[Article copies available for a fee from The Haworth Document Delivery Service: 1-800-HAWORTH. E-mail address: <docdelivery@haworthpress.com> Website: <http://www.HaworthPress.com> © 2006 by The Haworth Press, Inc. All rights reserved.]*

KEYWORDS. Welfare, welfare reform, single parents, comparative welfare policy

---

Martin Evans, PhD, is Senior Research Fellow, Centre for Analysis of Social Policy, University of Bath, Claverton Down, BATH BA2 7AY United Kingdom (E-mail: m.evans@bath.ac.uk). Jane Millar, PhD, is Professor of Social Policy, University of Bath, United Kingdom (E-mail: j.i.millar@bath.ac.uk).

[Haworth co-indexing entry note]: "Welfare to Work in the United Kingdom." Evans, Martin, and Jane Millar. Co-published simultaneously in *Journal of Policy Practice* (The Haworth Press, Inc.) Vol. 5, No. 2/3, 2006, pp. 61-76; and: *International Perspectives on Welfare to Work Policy* (ed: Richard Hoefer, and James Midgley) The Haworth Press, Inc., 2006, pp. 61-76. Single or multiple copies of this article are available for a fee from The Haworth Document Delivery Service [1-800-HAWORTH, 9:00 a.m. - 5:00 p.m. (EST). E-mail address: docdelivery@ haworthpress.com].

doi:10.1300/J508v05n02_05

INTRODUCTION AND CONTEXT

Britain and America are, once again, two nations separated by the same language when it comes to discussion of this commonly named policy area, welfare to work. We use many of the same key words but in a very different policy context. This includes some fundamental systemic differences. First, Tony Blair's Government since 1997 has undertaken a program of "Welfare Reform," as in the US. But the UK version includes a wide-ranging review of all systems of income transfers and is thus far more comprehensive than the 1996 Personal Responsibility and Work Opportunity Reconciliation Act and its antecedents. It includes the equivalent programs to Social Security, Unemployment Insurance, and SSI, as well as public assistance. Second, the UK's wider review of income transfers reflects in part a far more comprehensive system of coverage in the UK, which still maintains a national social assistance safety net for everyone aged over 18, irrespective of status. Additionally, there is a parallel national system of means-tested housing allowances and local taxation relief. The tax-funded National Health System provides both primary and secondary health care free at the point of access and thus avoids the need for means-tested Medicare and Medicaid. Third, the UK system is centralised and uniform, with no equivalent State-based differences, although there are local pilots and programs of various types operating in some localities.

Our approach is to navigate through such contextual differences by concentrating on the shared UK-US policy concern for single mothers, who are called "lone parents" in the UK. (Although this means we are focusing on just one of the groups targeted in the reform process, interested readers are referred to Walker and Wiseman [2003] for a more comprehensive account of the reform process in the UK). Our target audience is the American social work community who, as in the UK, mostly work for local government (Local Authorities in the UK) and do not have direct involvement in "welfare."

UK POLICY GOALS

The policy goals for lone parents are part of a wider set of systemic changes to employment, child-care and income maintenance programs that operate across the whole working age population. Over the 1980s and 1990s, there was a rising divide between work-rich and work-poor households despite continued structural changes to programs that focused on the "unemployed." Numbers of unemployed fluctuated with the economic cycle but across cycles the numbers of inactive people grew–either because of incapacity or through child caring responsibilities, effectively lone parents. This led to a growing polarisation between workless and work-rich households (Gregg and Wadsworth, 2003). Over the same period and as a consequence, poverty and child poverty increased greatly.

The government has therefore identified two key–and interrelated–policy goals. The first is to increase employment by reducing worklessness rather than just focusing on unemployment. This has led to a range of active labor market programs called "New Deals" that not only give increased resources to young and long-term unemployed but also extend such programs for the first time in the UK to lone parents and disabled people. Additionally, the need to increase employment of parents gave rise to the National Child Care Strategy and the expansion of "family-friendly" employment measures. Geographic concentrations of worklessness gave rise to a range of area-based programs.

The second major goal is to "end child poverty." Tony Blair announced in October 1999 that child poverty would be eliminated within a generation. This commitment has now been operationalised through intermediary targets: quartering child poverty by 2005, halving it by 2010 and ending it by 2020; and through the setting of poverty targets, all based on relative income measures and more generous than the US official poverty measure. The short-term policy instruments have been through increases in the generosity of children's benefits in social assistance (making welfare more generous) but also through more generous in-work payments to ensure that the mixture of employment (predominantly part-time for mothers) and tax credits–and for some, child support payments–combine together to substantially lift the incomes of families with children. Employment has the central role in the strategy for ending child poverty.

LONE PARENTS IN THE UK

Lone parents are defined as anyone with children under the age of 16 who has no co-resident partner. In this instance, the difference in terminology is important as the UK has no welfare policy concern with marital status, and thus single mothers and separated and divorced mothers are defined by their family composition only. Most lone parents (80%) are divorced or separated women. Lone parents are 26% of all families with children and have around 25% of all children (DWP, 2005a). However, 47% of lone-parent families live in poverty (measured as individuals below 60% of median equivalized after-housing-cost income) compared with 20% of couples with children. Twenty-eight percent of British children live in poverty but this risk of poverty rises to 74% with non-working lone parents (DWP, 2005a). This poverty is much more likely to be persistent. The employment rate for lone parents is around 55% which, compared to partnered mothers of around 71%, is far lower (House of Commons Work and Pensions Committee, 2004). Around 800,000 lone parents claim Income Support, the equivalent of US welfare and this represents around 44% of all lone parents (own calculations from DWP, 2005a; DWP, 2005c).

Public attitudes to state support for non-working lone parents remain generally positive, especially support for those with preschool children to choose whether or not to take up paid work (Millar, 2003). Income Support for these lone parents is paid without any obligation to work or seek work, until the youngest child reaches the age of 16. Employment is associated with two thirds of exits from low income for lone parents, and the risk of child poverty for lone parents in part-time employment falls to 27% (from 74% if not working) and falls further to 9% for full-time work (House of Commons Work and Pensions Committee, 2004).

PROMOTING LONE-PARENT EMPLOYMENT AND REDUCING POVERTY

The importance of employment in reducing lone-parent poverty has led the UK Government to set a target of a 70% lone-parent employment rate by 2010. To achieve this there have been a number of specific initiatives intended to increase financial incentives to work. These "make work pay" policies have included the introduction for the first time in the UK of a National Minimum Wage alongside a reduction in tax and social insurance costs of low-paid work. From April 2003, the child portions of Income Support were integrated with child support from tax credits into a new unified Child Tax Credit. Additionally, a working tax credit can be paid to those with low earnings. For lone parents part-time work is encouraged with a dividing line at 16 hours of employment a week. At this point the system pivots and cuts off entitlement to out-of-work Income Support and instead pays a Working Tax-Credit to lift income levels considerably at the margins of welfare and work. In April 2004, a lone parent with a single child aged less than 11 would receive about £117 per week in basic support, and would also have her rent and local taxation paid in addition. If she works for the minimum wage for just 16 hours a week she has a net income (after her rent is paid) of around £157, a substantial 40% increase in income. Of the total income in work, about a third comes from wages with the rest being made up of tax credits and other means-tested benefits. It must be stressed that tax credits in the UK are all available concurrently with earnings and no one has to wait until the end-of-year tax filing to receive payment. This makes the financial gains of work immediate and recognisably so in most cases. Indeed, research showed that most out-of-work lone parents sought to gain around £40 a week from entering employment (Lessof et al., 2003) and the current scheme almost meets this.

Of course, the actual financial situation of the family in work depends on a number of individual factors, including wages, child-care costs, transport costs, other work-related expenses, housing costs and child-support payments (Harries and Woodfield, 2002; Farrell and O'Connor, 2003; Woodland et al., 2003; Graham et al., 2005). Some families are not receiving the tax credits to which they are entitled and there have been problems with ensuring smooth payments of these tax credits (Citizen's Advice Bureau, 2005; National Audit Office, 2005). The child care tax credit only pays a portion of the costs of registered care, so is not received by all families who are paying for care. Being in work may also place other pressures on lone parents, including lack of time and difficulties in managing child care (Skinner, 2003; Bell et al., 2005). Many lone mothers who do work are in service-sector jobs, often quite low paid, and so work itself may be stressful and/or boring and repetitive. So, although families are usually financially better-off in work, this may not always be the case and they may not feel that they are much better-off when they take all these factors into account (Millar, 2005).

Lone-parent families can also face very high marginal tax rates in work. Apart from Child Benefit, which is paid to all families with children regardless of income level, in-work financial support is income-tested. The withdrawal of tax credits as income rises, alongside liabilities for tax and national insurance payments, can give rise to effective marginal tax rates of 70% to 85%. This is a disincentive to additional earners entering or remaining in the labor market and both studies of EITC and British antecedents to these Tax Credits have shown such means-tested in-work support most directly benefits single-earner families such as lone parents (see Blundell et al., 1998; Meyer and Rosenbaum, 2001, for instance).

In addition to "making work pay," the National Child-care Strategy has also improved provision of child-care places, with new child-care places for 1.6 million children by the end of 2003 and plans to increase to over two million places by 2006 (DWP, 2004b). However, the main financial subsidy for childcare comes in the form of an in-work tax credit which only pays up to 70% of weekly costs and is subject to a maximum level. The rest of the cost must be met by the lone parents themselves, which can be difficult if wages are low. Moreover, ensuring that child-care supply matches low-paid working mothers' requirements in terms of location, quality and quantity is still problematic, and area-based targeting of child-care supply to low-income neighbourhoods has also occurred. However, many lone parents choose to work part-time to minimise child-care costs as well as to fit employment around school hours.

At the same time as in-work support has increased, there have also been increases to child elements in out-of-work Income Support, now restructured as Child Tax Credit. Figure 1 shows how far the increases in generosity of these out-of-work payments have affected different types of families with children alongside changes in generosity of in-work pay-

FIGURE 1. Real Increases (Percent) in Value of UK Transfers for Children 1997-2003

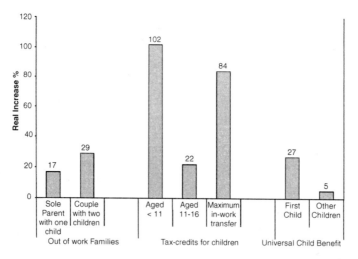

Source: Derived from Hills (2004), Table 9.1.

ments. The substantial increases in real generosity have been focused on young children aged under 11 in non-working families, and for all families with some paid work. However, for families out-of-work, the large increases in real terms in child components of their transfers is offset by no real increases to the amounts for adults. This means that while support for children under 11 has risen by 102%, when these children are placed alongside their parents, the increase is far less–17% for a sole parent and 29% for a couple with two such children. At the same time, universal benefits for the first child have also risen by 27%. The combined impact is thus to raise incomes in real terms by at least one-sixth for families out-of-work but to also improve incentives to work by large increases in the level of in-work support.

Overall, the combination of in-work tax credits (the pre-2003 programs), the National Minimum Wage and other aspects of reform have been estimated to increase lone-parent employment by seven percentage points–mainly though taking up part-time work (Gregg and Harkness, 2003). This has been achieved alongside fall in the poverty rates for all lone parents, not just those in work. Thus, unlike much of the similar increase in employment in the USA, the improvements for working lone parents have not been offset by higher poverty risks for those lone parents that remain out of work. Figure 2 shows the changes in poverty rates from 1996-97 to 2002-03.

Figure 2 shows that there is an almost unambiguous improvement on the most difficult of relative poverty measures (after housing costs) for all families with children, the only exception being couples who are not in work–a reflection of their income being in a majority made up of adult allowances for social assistance that have not been increased beyond price-inflation. Overall poverty for all children has fallen by 18% with greatest falls in poverty in larger families and in part-time working families (either lone parent or couple families). But even poverty for lone parents who do not work has fallen by 7%.

Survey evidence also shows, and again provides a distinct and counter-view from the evidence from the Survey of American Families in the USA (Zedlewski et al., 2002, for instance), that hardship for lone parent families, in and out of work, has fallen. Table 1 shows that a variety of measures of material deprivation and financial stress have fallen over the period of reform. UK welfare reform has delivered employment gains without the profile of hardship given by much of the US evidence.

FIGURE 2. Changes in Child Poverty by Family Type and Employment 1996/7 to 2002/3

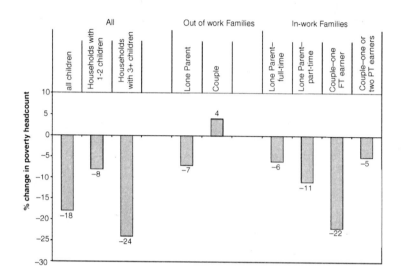

Notes: Proportional change in rates of after housing costs income measure.
Source: Derived from Stewart (2005), Table 7.3, based on data from the *Households Below Average Income Series.*

TABLE 1. Lone Parents; Material Deprivation and Selected Financial Stress Indicators: (Percent that Cannot Afford the Item)

	1999	2000	2001	2002
New, not second-hand clothes for family when needed	41%	35%	28%	25%
Best outfit for children	20	19	15	13
Celebration with presents on special occasions	27	23	17	14
Money for trips, holidays and outings	59	52	46	41
One week holiday away	74	69	62	58
Problems with debts most of the time	15	13	10	12
Run out of money before the end of the week/month	27	24	21	19
Worry about money almost always	45	38	33	30
Never has money left over	48	40	34	17

Source: Derived from list of material deprivation indicators in McKay and Collard (2003), Table 7.1.

NEW DEAL FOR LONE PARENTS

Alongside the policies to increase the pull of lone parents into work by making work pay, there have also been active labor market programs, which can be seen as accompanying "push" factors. This is an area where there is substantial difference between the US and the UK versions of welfare to work programs. British programs can be seen as persuasive and information-based, as a gentle prod, when compared to the erosion of entitlement and increase in mandation and sanctions that have occurred since PWRORA in the USA.

At the heart of the initiative is The New Deal for Lone Parents (NDLP), a voluntary program that primarily offers one-to-one advice and assistance in getting a job. NDLP is available to all lone parents claiming Income Support and has even been extended to those other lone parents who work less than 16 hours a week, although take-up by this latter group is very low. It is a voluntary program that consists of one or more meetings with a dedicated "personal advisor." Since it began in 1998, it has had a total caseload of over 940,000, which translates into around 680,000 individuals, as some people have been in the program more than once (DWP, 2005b). Around 365,000 job entries have resulted (DWP, 2005b).

In the early years of the program, entry was largely through invitation and self-referral and overall take-up rates were low, around 6% of the total stock of lone parents at any point in time. However, from 2001, there has been an introduction of mandatory employment orientation interviews as a part of a claim for Income Support and at regular intervals during a claim. These Work-Focused Interviews (WFIs) were introduced for all new claimants and rolled out over time for existing claimants, and are primarily about information giving and sharing concerning employment plans and opportunities. The mandatory requirement is to attend and take part in the interview; there is no mandation on action following a WFI. But WFIs have increased up-take of NDLP and are often delivered by the same personal advisor. The take-up of NDLP has risen to around 10% as a result, and new and recent lone parent claimants are particularly likely to agree to take part in the NDLP (Evans et al., 2003).

The role of, and work done, by Personal Advisers (PAs) is the crucial factor in NDLP delivery. They not only offer individually tailored advice to support lone parents into employment by finding employment opportunities from the electronic job database, but also assist and support lone parents in claiming in-work and transition benefits. They thus fill both entitlement and employment roles–ensuring that Income Support is paid when lone parents make a claim (there is no equivalent to US diversion approaches in the UK) and ensuring that in-work benefits and help with transitional support are claimed and paid as the lone parent moves into work. PAs thus have to establish and maintain a wide knowledge of local labor market information and link to local child-care information, and this information is all provided in one location (the network of local "Jobcentre Plus" offices).

The PAs' "toolkit" includes financial planning tools to help lone parents think through and plan changes in income sources and frequency. One element of this has proved to be extremely popular with lone parents, the "better-off" calculation, which enables the PA to demonstrate the likely gains to employment from either a theoretical job or an actual job offer that is in front of her. A lone parent's out-of-work claim will be composed of three elements, Child Tax Credit, which does not change, but also Income Support and Housing Benefits that will change when work starts. The PA helps to ensure that transitional financial help available from these benefits to "run-on" during the first weeks of employment is in place. Additionally, to meet one-off needs, the PA has an Adviser Discretionary Fund that can meet up to £300 of costs associated with returning to work–often up-front deposits for childcare, or travel season tickets, clothes or other items. Finally, the other element of the financial planning assistance is help completing tax credit claim forms together with an expedited claim service to ensure that payments in work occur as soon as is practicable.

The PA can assist with several tasks, such as a test trading period for lone parents who want to enter into self-employment, setting up limited training, and assisting with childcare and travel costs for part-time work (under 16 hours per week) for a limited period. All of these financial and planning elements of the PAs' job are in addition to their skills in job search assistance.

NDLP is a work-first program, and it shares this with the vast majority of US interventions. There is little opportunity to train or obtain education through NDLP. Although access to training programs has improved over time, such training is only for low-level vocational skills. The evaluation of NDLP surveyed participants to find out what happened during meetings with their PA. As one would expect from a voluntary program where some participants are "testing the water" there was not a 100% work focus. Table 2 shows the percentages of participants who reported different subjects covered in their meetings with Personal Advisers.

TABLE 2. The Content of PA Meetings in NDLP

% of Participants Reporting	Subject Covered
Employment Focus	
64%	work in general
55%	finding work
45%	help with vacancies
18%	help with job applications
11%	self-employment
Finance	
85%	had "better off calculations"
62%	advice on benefits
35%	help to fill in claim forms
Other	
58%	discussed childcare
27%	had help finding childcare
45%	discussed training
27%	had help finding training

Source: Derived from Lessof et al., 2003, Tables 4.3.1 to 4.3.4.

EVALUATION OF NDLP

There has been a very large investment in evaluation of NDLP along-side the other New Deal programs and other changes in delivery of employment and income transfer programs in Britain (Walker, 2004). The evaluation of NDLP has been both qualitative and quantitative (Evans et al., 2003) and we address these streams of evidence in turn. Most who take part are positive about the program and Personal Advisers are very highly regarded for both the help that is offered and their attitude and approach. Most participants say that everything they wanted was covered by the program, but the absence of in-built child care and training elements was perceived as a weakness. Informal outcomes have been found to be important with confidence building and the breaking down of isolation for lone parents, often stuck in the home, a major issue in improving well-being as well as employability and work orientation.

Qualitative evidence from lone parents who have recently entered work gives an indication of how successful NDLP can be to an individual: "Yes, I did go to a fantastic lady. . . with the job centre, and she was the one that helped me, worked out the tax credit, all my benefits and she got me some shoes . . . helped me with the process of filling in the forms . . . [I was] hoping that I wasn't going to have some time when I wasn't being paid . . . Which is where my lone parent adviser came in, she was great. Anything that went awry, she helped me through . . . It was quick . . . the right payment . . . it's all been absolutely fine" (Millar, 2005).

However, in measuring the quantitative impact of the program, its voluntary nature has made formal estimates of additionality difficult to establish. Take-up is still an issue and the success at getting participants into work is partly due to the most work-ready and motivated coming forward. In order to account for such selection bias a special survey was commissioned in which it was hoped to collect data on motivation and other aspects of attitudes that would enable participants and non-participants in the program to be accurately matched using propensity score methodology (Lessof et al., 2003). The results from this survey and the matching of participants to "identical" non-participants produced unexpectedly high impacts considering the nature of the program, low-cost face-to-face interview(s) with little use of costly elements such as child care, employment options, or full-time training courses that are used for more traditional unemployed target groups. Estimated additionality on work entry was 55% with a 25 percentage point difference in exits from Income Support between the participants and their matched control group. There is some argument as to whether selection bias has been properly controlled for and there have been a number of econometric studies to assess the methodology, but even so the program is found to have significant impacts that remain. In terms of cost effectiveness, the low costs of the program ensure that it remains cost-effective even if net additionality levels fall considerably (Evans et al., 2003).

Part of the success of the program has been due to the accompanying macro-economic and policy environment. The UK has had the longest period of sustained economic growth for 200 years, and this continued through the early 2000s. Accompanying NDLP have been the improvements in generosity of in-work support payments discussed earlier. The program has thus been able to take a self-selected group of lone parents and lever-in generous in-work supplements and an emerging growth in child-care provision at a time when demand for part-time low-skilled work was booming.

FINAL THOUGHTS

It is clear from our description that the common transatlantic phrase "welfare to work" hides clear and huge differences in both policy context and content. This is a clear warning about the need to avoid simple, or simplistic, comparisons based on text or rhetoric alone. Despite what appears to be a common and evolving consensus from the OECD and across other welfare states about the role of activation and employment programs for lone parents, these differences, between what may be interpreted as exemplars of the Anglo-Saxon model, far outweigh their harmonised rhetoric. Just because we are singing from the same hymn sheet doesn't mean we are singing in unison.

But the issues for Britain go far beyond the rhetoric because there are still unresolved issues for policy on lone-parent employment. There is significant cycling between welfare and work (Evans, Harkness, and Ortiz, 2004) with accompanying uncertainty about how to ensure better retention and advancement in work. The role of Personal Advisers has always involved in-work support after leaving welfare but much of this has been to assist further with claims for in-work benefits. There is currently in place an experimental demonstration plan to evaluate models of in-work support to encourage retention and advancement, but results are not due for two years or more and in the meantime there is continued discussion of the need for mentoring.

Furthermore, although lone-parent employment rates are steadily rising, they are not yet rising fast enough to reach the 70% target by 2010. The options are somewhat limited. Greater use of mandation to make people enter the program or work risks undermining the very things that make the program work as it would mean a shift in focus towards those lone parents who are not already at the margins of work. This would result in a bigger and more reluctant caseload with more complex needs, higher costs and lower aggregate average outcomes. Another option would be to lower the age of dependent children from 16 to, say, the age they enter secondary school at 12, and require work obligations from this group of lone mothers. This would have an effect on existing stocks of lone parents, but unlike the USA, such families would not fall out of entitlement altogether–as a result, they would merely shift into the unemployed group. They would still receive ongoing benefit support although they would be required to look for work, and take up suitable jobs. Failing that, the considerable proportion of lone parents with health problems would also find themselves in a different part of the system. One lesson from the New Deal is that the boundaries between target groups–the unemployed, the sick, and the lone parents–often hide levels of heterogeneity that cross boundaries. Further, these problems need individualised tailored responses rather than categorical ones. This lesson has been learned to some extent and more attention is now being placed on assessing needs and responses that go "beyond New Deal" group definitions. The really tough job will be to respond to the "hardest to serve" groups and to assist them into employment. Changes in definition or introduction of more mandation does not alter this.

As well as changing the push factors, there is also medium- to long-term uncertainty about the pull factors that attempt to ensure that employment and poverty prevention go hand in hand towards 2010 and 2020. The current consensus among independent analysts is that the UK Government will meet its aim of quartering child poverty by 2005 (Brewer, 2004; Sefton and Sutherland, 2005). However, the importance of a *relative* measure of poverty for the Government's target means that simply increasing benefits in line with prices (which is the current approach) will not be enough to maintain relative income levels over time. Thus, lone parents in low-paid part-time work will fall further behind median income growth and so not escape relative poverty (Evans and Eyre, 2004). Reaching 60 to 70% employment rates would fulfil one of the key policy goals but would not be enough in itself to eliminate child poverty in lone-parent families. More financial support for families with children, greater investment in child care, more support for working parents through "family friendly" employment practices–all this and more–will be required to meet the combination of employment increase and poverty elimination. The UK is thus not only attempting to "end welfare as we know it," as President Clinton famously labelled American welfare reform. To paraphrase Clinton, the UK aims to end child poverty as we know it and this means less focus on caseload reduction but more on fundamentally changing employment and income profiles of lone parents, without dismantling their entitlement to social assistance.

REFERENCES

Bell, A., Finch, N., La Valle, I., Sainsbury, R., & Skinner, C. (2005). *A Question of Balance: Lone Parents, childcare and work*. Department for Work and Pensions Research Report 230. Leeds: Corporate Document Services.

Blundell, R., Duncan, A., McCrae, J., & Meghir, C. (1998). *The Labour Market Impact of the Working Families Tax Credit. IFS Report to Bank of England Monetary Committee*. London: Institute for Fiscal Studies.

Brewer, M. (2004). *Will the Government Hit Its Child Poverty Target in 2004-05? Briefing Note Number 47.* London: Institute for Fiscal Studies.

Citizen's Advice Bureau (2005). *Money with Your Name on it? CAB Clients' Experience of Tax Credits.* London: Citizen's Advice Bureau.

Department for Work and Pensions (DWP) (2004a). *Tax Benefit Model Tables 2004.* London: Department for Work and Pensions.

Department for Work and Pensions (DWP) (2004b). *Departmental Report 2004.* London: Department for Work and Pensions. *http://www.dwp.gov.uk/publications/dwp/2004/dr04/execsum/home.asp*

Department for Work and Pensions (DWP) (2005a). *Households Below Average Income 1994-95-2003-04.* London: Department for Work and Pensions.

Department for Work and Pensions (DWP) (2005b). *New Deal for Lone Parents and Personal Advisor Meetings, Statistics to December 2004.* London: Department for Work and Pensions.

Department for Work and Pensions (DWP). (2005c). *Income Support Quarterly Statistical Enquiry.* London: Department for Work and Pensions.

Evans, M., Eyre, J., Millar, J., & Sarre, S. (2003). *New Deal for Lone Parents: Second Synthesis Report of the National Evaluation.* Sheffield: Department for Work and Pensions.

Evans, M., Harkness, S., & Ortiz, R. (2004). *Lone Parents Cycling Between Work and Benefits.* London: Department for Work and Pensions.

Evans, M., & Eyre, J. (2004). *The Opportunities of a Lifetime: A Model Lifetime Analysis of Current British Social Policy.* Bristol: Policy Press.

Farrell, C., & O'Connor, W. (2003). *Low-Income Families and Household Spending.* Department of Work and Pensions Research Report, No. 192, Leeds: Corporate Document Services.

Graham, J., Tennant, R., Huxley, M., & O'Connor, W. (2005) *The Role of Work in Low-Income Families with Children–A Longitudinal Qualitative Study.* Department of Work and Pensions Research Report, No. 245. Leeds: Corporate Document Services.

Gregg, P., & Harkness, S. (2003). Welfare reform and lone parents. In R. Dickens, P. Gregg, & J. Wadsworth (Eds.), *The Labour Market Under New Labour.* London: Palgrave, pp. 98-115.

Gregg, P., & Wadsworth, J. (2003). Workless households and the recovery. In R. Dickens, P. Gregg, & J. Wadsworth (Eds.), *The Labour Market Under New Labour.* London: Palgrave, pp. 32-39.

Harries, T., & Woodfield, K. (2002). *Easing the Transition into Work,* DWP Research Report, No. 175. Leeds: Corporate Document Services.

Hills, J. (2004). *Inequality and the State.* Oxford: Oxford University Press.

House of Commons Work and Pensions Committee (2004). *Second Report: Child Poverty in the UK (HC 85-1).* London: The Stationery Office.

Lessof, C., Miller, M., Phillips, M., Pickering, K., Purdon, S., & Hales, J. (2003). *New Deal for Lone Parents Evaluation: Findings from the Quantitative Survey.* Sheffield: Employment Service, WAE147.

McKay, S., & Collard, S. (2003). *Developing Deprivation Questions for the Family Resources Survey.* Bristol: Personal Finance Research Centre, University of Bristol.

Meyer, B., & Rosenbaum, D. (2001). Welfare, the Earned Income Tax Credit, and the labor supply of single mothers. *Quarterly Journal of Economics,* CXVI, 1063-1114.

Millar, J. (2003). The art of persuasion: The new deal for lone parents. In R.Walker & M. Wiseman (Eds.), *The Welfare We Want.* Bristol: Policy Press, pp. 115-142.

Millar, J. (2005). Making ends meet in paid work: Lone mothers, income packages and income risk. Unpublished paper presented at *Cash and care: A conference in memory of Sally Baldwin.* University of York, UK.

National Audit Office (2005). *Inland Revenue: Standard Report 2003-2004: Child and Working Tax Credits and Stamp Duty Land Tax.* London: National Audit Office.

Sefton, T., & Sutherland, H. (2005). Inequality and poverty under New Labour. In J. Hills & K. Stewart (Eds.), *A More Equal Society: New Labour, Poverty, Inequality and Social Exclusion.* Bristol: Policy Press, pp. 231-250.

Skinner, C. (2003). *Running around in circles: Coordinating Childcare, Education and Work,* Bristol: Policy Press/ Joseph Rowntree Foundation, Work and Family Series.

Stewart, K. (2005). Towards an equal start? Addressing childhood poverty and deprivation. In J. Hills & K. Stewart (Eds.), *A More Equal Society: New Labour, Poverty, Inequality and Social Exclusion.* Bristol: Policy Press, pp. 143-166.

Walker, R. (2004). Evaluation: Evidence for public policy. In A. Nolan & G. Wong (Eds.), *Evaluating Local Economic and Employment Development: How to Assess What Works Among Programmes and Policies.* Paris: OECD, pp. 63-111.

Walker, R., & Wiseman, M. (2003). *The Welfare We Want: The British Challenge for American Reform.* Bristol: Policy Press.

Woodland, S., Mandy, W., & Miller, M. (2003). *Easing the Transition into Work (part 2-client survey),* Department for Work and Pensions Research Report Number 186. Leeds: Corporate Document Services.

Zedlewski, S., Giannarelli, L., Morton, J., & Wheaton, L. (2002). *Extreme Poverty Rising, Existing Government Programs Could Do More.* Washington: Urban Institute Assessing New Federalism Program.

Social Inclusion as an Agenda
for Mental Health Social Work:
Getting a Whole Life?

Nick Gould

SUMMARY. Following New Labour's election to office in the UK in 1997, policy initiatives have proliferated relating to mental health. Much of this policy innovation emphasises the social dimensions of mental health and distress, with an emphasis on employment and social inclusion. Paradoxically, this modernization of the mental health agenda comes at a time when mental health social work is struggling to establish its role and contribution within recently integrated health and social services. The paper considers whether New Labour's flagship programme, *Mental Health and Social Exclusion*, constitutes a "New Deal" for mental health, and whether it provides a perspective that will help mental health social work to define its distinctive contribution to integrated services. *[Article copies available for a fee from The Haworth Document Delivery Service: 1-800-HAWORTH. E-mail address: <docdelivery@haworthpress.com> Website: <http://www.HaworthPress.com> © 2006 by The Haworth Press, Inc. All rights reserved.]*

KEYWORDS. Mental health policy, UK, New Labour

Nick Gould, PhD, is Professor of Social Work, Department of Social and Policy Sciences, University of Bath, Claverton Down, BATH BA2 7AY United Kingdom (E-mail: hssng@bath.ac.uk).

[Haworth co-indexing entry note]: "Social Inclusion as an Agenda for Mental Health Social Work: Getting a Whole Life?" Gould, Nick. Co-published simultaneously in *Journal of Policy Practice* (The Haworth Press, Inc.) Vol. 5, No. 2/3, 2006, pp. 77-90; and: *International Perspectives on Welfare to Work Policy* (ed: Richard Hoefer, and James Midgley) The Haworth Press, Inc., 2006, pp. 77-90. Single or multiple copies of this article are available for a fee from The Haworth Document Delivery Service [1-800-HAWORTH, 9:00 a.m. - 5:00 p.m. (EST). E-mail address: docdelivery@ haworthpress.com].

doi:10.1300/J508v05n02_06

INTRODUCTION

Since New Labour's election to office in 1997 there has been a surge of mental health policy initiatives designed to modernise mental health services. At the same time, wider invigoration of debates over social models of mental health are taking place, particularly the emergence of social inclusion as a core objective of UK mental health policy. In summer 2004 the Social Exclusion Unit's report *Mental Health and Social Exclusion* announced a programme of activities intended to increase social inclusion of people with mental health problems, with a significant role for implementation allocated to the social care sector. This has been contemporaneous with a comprehensive reconfiguration of the organisational position of mental health social work, which has been relocated from local authority social service departments into National Health Service trusts. Mental health social workers now find themselves managed within multidisciplinary team settings in which social care is a minority player.

A paradox seemingly characterises mental health social work in the English context. New Labour has championed mental health as a priority development area within the National Health Service. Furthermore, much of the policy framework for the modernization of mental health services emphasises the social dimension of mental health needs (Duggan et al., 2003). This would appear to offer an unprecedented opportunity for the assertion of the relevance and importance of social work to the multidisciplinary care of users of mental health services. However, despite this platform, there is substantial evidence showing a crisis of morale in mental health social work, with particular difficulties in adjusting to practice within integrated health and social care structures (Carpenter et al., 2003). A national survey conducted by the Institute of Psychiatry (Huxley, 2003) shows: social workers in mental health settings have higher stress levels than psychiatrists (measured by the General Health Questionnaire); a large percentage are planning to leave mental health as a specialty (20-25% have a strong or very strong desire to leave); an ageing work force (42% over 50) with problems of attracting young social workers. Recent qualitative studies illuminate some of the anxieties underlying this malaise: concerns that the integration of health and social services will marginalise the social work contribution and that social workers cannot articulate their distinct contribution to the multi-professional mix (Blinkhorn, 2003; Williams, 2003).

That there are agendas of social justice and social inequality in the mental health field is widely evidenced (see Social Exclusion Unit, 2003 for an overview). There is a raft of empirical evidence to show the acute social disadvantages of many people with mental health problems (Rogers & Pilgrim, 2003); even amongst people with disabilities they are relatively deprived. For example, adults with mental health problems have the lowest employment rate of any of the main groups of disabled people (Office for National Statistics, 2003). The number of people claiming sickness and disability benefits for mental health conditions is larger than the total number of unemployed people claiming Jobseeker's Allowance in England (Office for National Statistics, 2004). In an assessment of the national impact of the issues, a Sainsbury Centre for Mental Health report (2003) concluded that the total economic and social costs in England of mental distress are £77 billion a year. Various commentators have indicated that, given these factors, social inclusion represents an analytical perspective that should inform the development of mental health policy (Sayce, 2001; Huxley & Thornicroft, 2003; Repper & Perkins, 2003; Williams, 2003).

There has been a veritable blizzard of policy initiatives relating to mental health to appear since New Labour came to power in 1997. It has been calculated that in the first four years of office, 650 policy documents relating to mental health were published (*Community Care*, June 2004, 10-16). The keystone document has been the National Service Framework for Mental Health (NSF) in 1999, which–for adults of working age–sets a series of standards to be achieved within 10 years across health and social services (Department of Health, 1999). The first set of standards relate to the reduction of stigma and social exclusion. The NSF was accompanied by an additional funding allocation of £700m. to mental health services for the subsequent three years. The framework was shortly followed by the NHS National Plan that named mental health as one of the three priority areas for the health service (Department of Health, 2000).

The organisational framework for modernization of mental health services has been addressed through various new institutional arrangements. The task for leading modernization was entrusted to a purpose-created agency, the National Institute for Mental Health England (NIMHE) (Lelliott, 2002). The justification for this was that a unified organization with a national centre, led by the National Director for Mental Health, would most effectively coordinate support for reform through eight regional development centres. NIMHE sits alongside a complex constellation of actors with responsibilities for various performance aspects of mental health services, including: strategic health authorities; local implementation teams to take forward the NSF; primary care trusts with commissioning responsibilities for mental health services; the Commission for Healthcare Audit and Inspection; the Commission for Social Care Inspection which, along with the Audit Commission, reviews the social services element of mental health services; and patients' forums in every NHS and primary care trust to monitor and review services from a user perspective.

JOINING UP MENTAL HEALTH AND SOCIAL INCLUSION POLICY

Some commentators had latterly been concerned that despite all this activity, the seemingly emergent social dimensions of mental health policy and services were already in retreat (Goldie, 2003, 37). Concerns expressed include the fear that the National Service Framework, whilst establishing a platform for modernization, has drawn resources towards those aspects that are focused on clinical treatment, with less attention to the development of whole systems approaches that require close working across a wide range of agencies. Employment schemes, it was claimed, had particularly been downgraded by this shift towards treatment. So, the announcement in 2003 of a cross-departmental approach to social exclusion and mental health, led by the Office of the Deputy Prime Minister's Social Exclusion Unit, promised to rally activities that bolstered a social approach.

The subsequent report, *Mental Health and Social Exclusion* (Social Exclusion Unit, 2004), sets out a range of cross-departmental initiatives to coordinate activity to reduce the social exclusion of people with mental health problems. The initial consultation document outlined the remit of the project:

> The Social Exclusion Unit is undertaking a project to investigate how to reduce social exclusion among adults with mental health problems. The project will consider how to improve rates of employment, through support both in retaining and taking up work. It will also consider how to promote social participation and access to a broad range of services in the community. The project will then deliver a set of concrete recommendations designed to bring about real improvements in services, support and employment opportunities. (Social Exclusion Unit, 2003, 2)

The final report draws upon a process of broad consultation that included surveys of people with mental health problems, carers, health, social and voluntary service workers, local authorities, housing, employment and benefit services. The SEU also commissioned seven systematic reviews of relevant research, seven consultation events to identify views of users and carers, four local area research studies to capture an understanding of service delivery issues, and 50 visits to projects already addressing mental health and social exclusion issues.

The report's recommendations are supported by six general principles, that:

- Communities should accept that people with mental health problems are equal.
- People should receive the support they need before they reach crisis point.
- People should have genuine choices and a real say about what they do and the support they receive in order to achieve their potential.
- People should be helped to keep their jobs longer and return to employment faster, with real opportunities for career advancement.
- The importance of people's relationships, family and caring responsibilities should be recognised as well as access to basic resources including a decent home, and participation in social and leisure activities.
- Health and social care services should work in close partnership with employment and community services, with fair access regardless of ethnicity, gender, age or sexuality.

The report sets out a 27-point action plan to bring together government departments and agencies to improve outcomes for people with mental distress under six headings:

- *Stigma and discrimination*–a programme to challenge negative attitudes and promote awareness of people's rights. The report announces a £1.1 million programme to counter discrimination against people with mental health problems, including the development of educational materials, and support implementation of a proposed public sector duty to promote equal opportunities for disabled people.

- *The role of health and social care in tackling social exclusion*–implementing "evidence-based practice" in vocational services and enabling reintegration into the community; accessing an employment adviser; redesigning day services to promote social inclusion; better training for practitioners on social inclusion; reducing inequalities in access to services; and closer cooperation between mental health and criminal justice systems.
- *Employment*–better services for adults with mental health problems to find and retain work; pilot schemes to evaluate the use of specialist personal advisers to manage their condition in a work environment; more mental health training for Jobcentre Plus staff; consideration of improvements to linking rules and permitted work rules to support the transition from benefits to work; improved support for employers through the government's vocational rehabilitation framework.
- *Supporting families and community participation*–the report recognises the impact of mental health problems on the emotional development of children, and the effects on wider family and friends. In relation to community-based cultural and leisure facilities there is commitment expressed for increasing support to access education and training opportunities; strengthening the evidence-base to enable "wider roll-out of arts interventions": targeted family support to meet needs of parents with mental health problems and their children; and increased involvement of people with mental health problems in service design.
- *Basic needs*–new guidance to housing authorities on lettings and achieving stability for people with mental health problems; and better access to financial and legal advice, and affordable transport.
- *Implementation*–clear arrangements for leading the programme achieved through a cross-government team overseen by ministers; an independent advisory group to advise government on progress; local implementation to be supported by NIMHE; and better use of expertise in the voluntary and community sector.

Implementation will be monitored through annual reports collating a range of indicators drawn primarily from existing sources of information (SEU, 2004, 112), in most cases the Department of Health Psychiatric Morbidity Survey and the Labour Force Survey.

BUT IS IT SOCIAL INCLUSION AS WE KNOW IT?

A striking feature of the report is the absence of any definition of either social inclusion or social exclusion. Atkinson et al. (2002, 3) have argued that part of the rhetorical power of these terms indeed lies in their frequent lack of definition (who could be in favour of social exclusion?), though this threatens to undermine their analytical bite. The presumption seems to be that there is sufficient intuitive grasp of what social exclusion means to know which range of issues are implied, e.g., poverty, unemployment, low education, poor housing, incapacity to participate in social activities. However, this leaves us with difficulties precisely in judging the completeness of any analysis of social inclusion. At what point do we stop iterating the list of exclusions? It also tends to focus on outcomes but leaves unexamined the dynamics of the trajectories of social exclusion. Do the SEU's report headings relating to stigma, changes in health and social care services, employment, family and community participation, and access to basic services cover all the bases of a joined-up approach to tackling social exclusion?

The report certainly approaches social inclusion from a wider perspective than that of individual or household financial deprivation, and considers areas for social intervention such as stigma, housing, employment, participation in community activities, and access to services. Whether this builds to a holistic perspective is a more complicated issue, and comes up against some of the complexities besetting research into pathways of people with mental health problems. Ever since the seminal research by Faris and Dunham (1939) on mental illness and social class there have been major analytical problems in sifting the evidence between "drift" hypotheses which speculate that the onset of mental disorder produces downward social mobility, and "stress" hypotheses that the challenge of living in disadvantaged localities produces or amplifies mental distress. Correlational studies that lack longitudinal data are of little help in untangling these complexities. It may also be the case that we should not think of people with mental health problems as a generic category; the process of social exclusion varies between mental disorder and between individuals. For example, the seminal research of Brown and Harris (1978) illuminated the relationship between life events and onset of depression in working-class women. Recent qualitative research (Davidson, 2003) into the experiences of people with schizophrenia suggests some of the interactions between social factors and individual exclusion.

Exclusion is characterised not only by the depletion of personal resources, but also by lack of opportunity or capacity to connect with facilities or supports in the community. The latest approach to measuring of deprivation at a small area level ("super output areas") produced for the Office for National Statistics (2004) now contains indicators of mental illness and reinforces the known evidence about the spatial concentration of poor mental health in areas of multiple deprivation. Also, the King's Fund in conjunction with NIMHE has emphasised the need to make strategic links between community renewal initiatives and mental health (Cameron et al., 2003). However, social exclusion implies not only the geographical concentration of disadvantage, but also impoverishment of the quality and characteristics of relationships between individuals and their network, their social capital (Webber, 2005).

Whereas poverty research has tended to focus on identification of a meaningful threshold between being in or out of poverty, an implication of the discourse of social inclusion is that there is a point in the trajectory of becoming socially excluded of "no return"; a detachment from normative levels of social functioning that is so decisive as to mitigate against rehabilitation or reintegration (Room, 1999). Recent longitudinal research does show that some groups, including people with disabilities, are at greater risk of being socially excluded on a longer-term basis (Agulnik et al., 2002). Though disability has been identified as a generic risk factor and we have already commented on the prevalence of disadvantage amongst people with mental health problems, there is less discussion within the SEU report of the needs of people with chronic, long-term problems. Various commentators within the mental health community have registered concerns that service innovations being driven by the NSF focusing on early intervention, crisis intervention and other acute services are directing attention and resources from people whose difficulties are relatively chronic and long-term. There is also survey evidence that long-term mental health service users perceive themselves to be the "forgotten generation" in the modernization of mental health policy (Rethink, 2004).

A NEW DEAL FOR MENTAL HEALTH SOCIAL WORK?

So what are the implications of all this for social work? The emphasis on the centrality of employment to counter social exclusion presents a challenge for traditional British conceptualisations of the social work role (Jordan, 1984). Though multidimensional in its scope, the SEU report is permeated with references to the centrality of employment. Indeed, a recent report refers to it as "the Social Exclusion Unit's report on the employment of people with mental health problems" (Social Services Inspectorate, 2004, 32). This chimes strongly with the central thrust of New Labour social inclusion policy, that it is most effectively achieved through work, an objective pursued through a diverse range of New Deal programmes which prioritise reinsertion of socially excluded people into the labour market. Even when addressing issues such as modernization of day services or closer cooperation between health and social care, there are frequent references in the SEU report to preparation for employment as a justification for service improvement. Where then does the report sit alongside the various elements of New Deal policy? This should be of concern given a prominent assessment of New Deal projects that they are "less good at dealing with people with multiple problems and needs" (Millar, 2000, vi).

Dean (2003) has drawn a distinction between welfare to work policies that follow a "work first" model (as in the United States) prioritising labour market participation–on the grounds that any job is better than none–and the European "human capital" model which prioritises so-called "supply-side" capacities of individuals in the form of inculcating work-oriented attitudes and marketable skills and capacities. Dean has suggested that New Labour's model represents a classical British compromise: its activation policies have been implemented through national programmes that prioritise inserting unemployed people into the labour market as quickly as possible, but this is balanced by educational opportunities, training schemes and personal advice aimed at giving some enhancement to the employability of people from targeted groups such as disabled people or lone parents.

Mental Health and Social Exclusion reflects numerous aspects of the British New Deal model. Throughout the report there is prominence given to the challenge of finding and retaining paid work by people with mental health problems, supported by reference to the survey and consultation evidence that this is also considered a priority for service users. At the same time the report does not advocate the extension of any compulsions that already exist within the benefit system. But does it engage with the deeper impoverishment of the lives of many people with mental health problems, what Dean refers to as their "ontological needs" (2003, 441)? In Dean's words, what are needed are "life-first approaches," policies that recognise work as an important source of esteem and identity, but also acknowledge the basic struggle for some people to find meaning and direction in their lives. For many, their capacity to cope fluctuates significantly over long periods of time. As mentioned above, a survey by Rethink (2004), a leading UK mental health charity, found that the concentration of attention on young and acutely unwell people left behind an estimated 50,000 people who are regarded as medically "stable" but who are isolated and have a poor quality of life. Where they are able to engage with work they tend to be caught up in a "low pay-no pay" cycle, exposed to the most negative aspects of a "flexible" labour market. A social exclusion policy will offer little protection to people if there is not also attention given to protection from some of these risks.

Above all, a comprehensive social inclusion policy for mental health needs to be systemic. It will be difficult for implementation agencies to bring about reductions in social exclusion of people with mental health problems when other policies undercut the objectives of the SEU report. As examples of some of the present contradictions: at the same time that the implementation of the SEU report is getting underway, there is news that the same department, the Office of the Department of the Deputy Prime Minister, has announced a 7% cut in real terms over the next three years in the Supporting People budget, with accompanying clarification that services for people with mental health problems "were not appropriate for Supporting People funding" (Kumar, 2004). This is despite the fact that the number of people with mental health problems receiving Supporting People funding is identified as an indicator of progress in implementing the SEU report. Again, the Home Office continues to preside over rapid expansion of the prison population; August 2004 saw a record number of suicides in English prisons (Herbert, 2004), despite suicide reduction being a standard in the mental health NSF. Meanwhile, at the Department of Health, the second draft of the Mental Health Bill has been published which has drawn wide criticism for its enlargement of professional discretion in relation to coercive treatment of individuals. Despite some modifications from the first (2001) draft, it has been received immediately by the Director of the Mental Health Foundation as "a shameful step backwards" because of the effect of its broader definition of mental disorder on labelling and stigmatisation of people needing help from mental health services (Mental Health Foundation press release 8, September 2004).

New Labour has been described as "essentially ambiguous and Janus-faced," indicating the "often contradictory and conflicting traditions of social democracy, social conservatism, Thatcherism and pragmatism" (Lister, 2003, 438). Mental health policy is an exemplar of these contradictions: an espoused commitment to making mental health a priority accompanied by a raft of modernization initiatives that give social perspectives an unprecedented prominence in recent times. But this operates against a wider range of governmental policy that impacts the relative disadvantage of people with mental health problems. Whether these can be translated into real gains for social inclusion and justice will depend not only upon achievement of the targets surfaced by the *Mental Health and Social Exclusion* report, important and welcome as they are, but whether a wider public health perspective can emerge that sees social inclusion for mental health as integral to economic and social policy in their widest conceptions.

IMPLICATIONS FOR SOCIAL WORK PRACTICE

We have argued that there is a reemergence of social perspectives in mental health, and that although the arguments are diverse, overall they indicate an outlook that differs in a number of respects from earlier anti-psychiatry and social constructionist perspectives. They emerge against a backdrop of institutional change that, within a broad consensus on the undesirability of confinement in large institutions, nevertheless has followed diverging pathways in developing mental health services within welfare regimes. They will continue to respond to a range of pressures related to globalization that have mental health implications, albeit those responses will be shaped by local circumstances and path dependencies.

This paper has suggested that emergent social models or perspectives present some "middle-range" principles that need to inform mental health social work practice. The quality of life desired by people in mental distress is multifaceted and goes beyond the effects of compliance with pharmacological interventions. Many of the problems experienced by people in mental distress are produced by the exclusionary tendencies of social institutions rather than the inherent limitations of those individuals. This perspective has been extensively developed within disability theory but needs continuing elaboration in the context of mental health (Beresford, 2002). Thus, the operation of power is critical in understanding the dynamics of mental health; social work has an established tradition of working in anti-discriminatory and anti-oppressive ways–this is a contribution that can be made to the wider development of mental health practice in multidisciplinary settings. Rediscovery of the community and locality as a context within which mental health and distress are experienced also reasserts community development as a legitimate aspect of social work practice, alongside individual psychosocial interventions.

But if social work is to take social inclusion of people in mental distress seriously as a framework for practice, then some broadening of our view of the scope of social work is overdue. Taking Hill's (2002) multidimensional model of social inclusion, service users need to be seen in the round as producers, consumers, participants and social actors, not just as recipients of services. In relation to production it involves closer involvement in brokerage of job finding and retention, an area that has not only been outside the training and education of British social workers, but also traditionally disdained as beyond the remit of therapeutic orientations to professional practice. As Jordan has commented, social work will need to "take a broader view of its remit, to include economic activity, social regeneration, community work and many projects and units that do not at present think of themselves in its terms" (Jordan, 2000). If social work does not engage in these arenas, then the likelihood is that its role in relation to social exclusion will be colonised by other newly emerging occupational groups, such as the Department of Work and Pension's "personal advisers" within government employment agencies, who will have little training in mental health or social interventions.

Likewise, it requires a more proactive engagement with radical policy initiatives that empower people as commissioners of their own services, particularly direct payments (a recent UK innovation giving service users their own budget to purchase services directly). The allocation of monetary benefits has deep associations within the culture of British social work with Speenhamland and Poor Law traditions; both radical and therapeutic perspectives in social work have eschewed the co-optation of social workers as gatekeepers of systems that pauperise and disempower service users. However, direct payments require social workers to reassess, at least in respect to this provision, their traditional disdain for allocation of money. If empowerment and recovery are to be taken seriously, then social work has to engage with direct payments as a strategy for partnership and enfranchisement of service users as commissioners of their own services.

Seen as opportunities, rather than threats, the emerging framework of social inclusion policy creates a platform for mental health social work that could reassert its contribution to integrated multi-professional services. Nevertheless, we should be cautious in seeing social inclusion policy, as currently formulated, as a complete panacea for the difficulties experienced by people in mental distress. As we have seen, there remains a range of policy areas, not least in relation to the criminal justice system and mental health law, where there is still much "joining up" to be done.

REFERENCES

Agulnik, P., Burchardt, T., & Evans, M. (2002). Response and prevention in the British welfare state. In J. Hills, J. Le Grand, & D. Piachaud (Eds.), *Understanding Social Exclusion.* Oxford: Oxford University Press, pp. 155-177.

Atkinson, T., Cantillon, B., Marlier, E., & Nolan, B. (2002). *Social Indicators: The EU and Social Inclusion.* Oxford: Oxford University Press.

Beresford, P. (2002). Thinking about "mental health": Towards a social model. *Journal of Mental Health, 11*(6), 581-584.

Bhui, K., Stansfeld, S., Hull, S., Priebe, S., & Mole, F. (2004). Ethnic variation–Pathways to and use of specialist mental health services in the UK. *British Journal of Psychiatry, 182,* 105-116.

Blinkhorn, M. (2004). *Social Worker: Leading Roles in Mental Health.* Durham: Northern Centre for Mental Health.

Brown, G., & Harris, T. (1978). *Social Origins of Depression.* London: Tavistock Publications.

Burchardt, T., Le Grand, J., & Piachaud, D. (2002). Degrees of exclusion: Developing a dynamic, multidimensional measure. In J. Hills, J. Le Grand, & D. Piachaud (Eds.), *Understanding Social Exclusion.* Oxford: Oxford University Press, pp. 30-43.

Cameron, M., Edmans, T., Greatley, A., & Morris, D. (2003). *Community Renewal and Mental Health: Strengthening the Links.* London: King's Fund and NIMHE.

Carpenter, J., Schneider, J., Brandon, B., & Wooff, D. (2003). Working in multidisciplinary community mental health teams: The impact on social workers and health professionals of integrated mental health care. *British Journal of Social Work, 33,* 1081-1103.

Davidson, L. (2003). *Living Outside Mental Illness: Qualitative Studies of Recovery in Schizophrenia.* New York: New York Press.

Dean, H. (2003). Re-conceptualising welfare to work for people with multiple problems and needs. *Journal of Social Policy, 32*(3), 441-459.

Department of Health (1999). *A National Service Framework for Mental Health.* London: Stationery Office.

Department of Health (2000). *The National Plan.* London: Stationery Office.

Duggan, M. with Cooper, A., & Foster, J. (2003). *Modernising the Social Model in Mental Health, Social Perspectives Network Paper 1.* Available from www.spn.org.uk.

Faris, R., & Dunham, H. (1939). *Mental Disorders in Urban Areas.* Chicago: University of Chicago Press.

Herbert, I. (2004). Prisoner suicides rise to record level in overcrowded jails. *The Independent,* September 4, 2004, 16.

Hills, J., Le Grand, J., & Piachaud, D. (Eds) (2002). *Understanding Social Exclusion.* Oxford: Oxford University Press.

Huxley, P., & Thornicroft, G. (2003). Social inclusion, social quality and mental illness. *British Journal of Psychiatry, 182,* 289-290.

Jordan, B. (1984). *An Invitation to Social Work.* Oxford: Martin Robertson.

Jordan, B., & Jordan, C. (2000). *Social Work and the Third Way: Tough Love as Social Policy.* London: Sage Publications.

Millar, J. (2000). *Keeping Track of Welfare Reform: The New Deal Programmes.* York: Joseph Rowntree Foundation.

Office for National Statistics (2003). *Labour Force Survey August 2003.* London: Office for National Statistics.

Office for National Statistics (2004). *Labour Market Statistics May 2004.* London: Office for National Statistics.

Repper, J., & Perkins, J. (2003). *Social Inclusion and Recovery: A Model for Mental Health Practice.* Edinburgh: Bailliere Tindall.

Rethink (2004). *Lost and Found: Voices from the Forgotten Generation.* London: Rethink.

Rogers, A., & Pilgrim, D. (2003). *Mental Health and Inequality.* Basingstoke: Palgrave Macmillan.

Room, G. (1999). Social exclusion, solidarity and the challenge of globalization. *International Journal of Social Welfare, 8,* 166-174.

Sainsbury Centre for Mental Health (2003). *Economic and Social Costs of Mental Illness in England.* London: Sainsbury Centre for Mental Health.

Sayce, L. (2001). Social inclusion and mental health. *Psychiatric Bulletin, 25*(4), 121-123.

Social Exclusion Unit (2004). *Mental Health and Social Exclusion.* London: Office of the Deputy Prime Minister.

Social Services Inspectorate (2004). *Treated as People: An Overview of Mental Health Services from a Social Care Perspective, 2002-04.* London: SSI.

Webber, M. (2005). Social capital and mental health. In J. Tew (Ed.), *Social Perspectives in Mental Health.* London: Jessica Kingsley.

Williams, C. (2003). *From Social Care to Social Inclusion.* York: Northern Development Centre.

Helping People with Learning Difficulties into Paid Employment: Will UK Social Workers Use the Available Welfare to Work System?

Mark Baldwin

SUMMARY. Welfare to work policies have developed partly from policy rhetoric that argues employment as the best way of ensuring social inclusion for marginalised groups. In the United Kingdom, welfare to work policies for disabled people have developed within an enabling rather than a mandatory system, although organisation and practice have lagged behind. This article explores policies that provide this enabling context for facilitating the transition of people with learning difficulties from benefits to paid employment. It also explores the role of social workers, examining the degree to which their practice reflects the empowering rhetoric of the policy framework and of contemporary social work values. *[Article copies available for a fee from The Haworth Document Delivery Service: 1-800-HAWORTH. E-mail address: <docdelivery@haworthpress.com> Website: <http://www.HaworthPress.com> © 2006 by The Haworth Press, Inc. All rights reserved.]*

Mark Baldwin, PhD, is Senior Lecturer in Social Work, University of Bath, Claverton Down, BATH BA2 7AY United Kingdom (E-mail: m.j.baldwin@bath.ac.uk).

[Haworth co-indexing entry note]: "Helping People with Learning Difficulties into Paid Employment: Will UK Social Workers Use the Available Welfare to Work System?" Baldwin, Mark. Co-published simultaneously in *Journal of Policy Practice* (The Haworth Press, Inc.) Vol. 5, No. 2/3, 2006, pp. 91-107; and: *International Perspectives on Welfare to Work Policy* (ed: Richard Hoefer, and James Midgley) The Haworth Press, Inc., 2006, pp. 91-107. Single or multiple copies of this article are available for a fee from The Haworth Document Delivery Service [1-800-HAWORTH, 9:00 a.m. - 5:00 p.m. (EST). E-mail address: docdelivery@haworthpress.com].

Available online at http://www.haworthpress.com/web/JPP
© 2006 by The Haworth Press, Inc. All rights reserved.
doi:10.1300/J508v05n02_07

91

KEYWORDS. Welfare to work, social inclusion, disability, policy implementation, social work practice

INTRODUCTION

There is a widespread view in policy circles in Europe, the USA and Australia that work is the key to achieving social inclusion for marginalised people such as those who are disabled. For example, the Social Exclusion Unit within the Office of the Deputy Prime Minister in the UK's New Labour government expressly argues the case for focusing policy development on getting people into work as the key to their inclusion (Office of the Deputy Prime Minister, 2003). I do not intend to get into the debate on the nature of social exclusion as a concept, but it is important to note the primacy of this policy intention and the practice implications that follow from it. Are disabled people included in the policy framework for achieving this aim? If so, how well is the policy working? Inasmuch as social workers are key practitioners assisting disabled people, what part are they playing in the process of inclusion? These are the questions that this article will address, in relation to policy and practice in the UK, and focused on people who are disabled by general responses to their learning difficulty (n.b. "learning difficulty" is the preferred phrase for self-advocates in the UK. The British Government refers to "learning disabilities." Other countries use phrases such as intellectual impairment. I will use the phrase preferred by disabled people in the UK).

Whilst the UK government wants to be positive about this policy initiative, it is the case that there is considerable disquiet about a work-based route to inclusion generally (Clegg, 2005), as well as specific problems for disabled people (Levitas, 1998). On the latter issue there are dangers of exploitation of disabled people at the bottom of the employment market. Most work that has been provided for people with learning difficulties has been menial and often unpaid (Department of Health, 2001), and seen as occupation for therapeutic purposes rather than paid employment. The policy of seeing work as the main route to social inclusion also has the disadvantage of further marginalisation for those who cannot engage in paid work (Levitas, 1998), because of the severity of their difficulties–either physical or learning. The policy could, therefore, produce an increasingly smaller residue of people who were not able to engage in paid work and would, therefore, remain socially excluded.

As the policy unfolds, however, people with learning difficulties who have been given the opportunity to understand that work might be a possibility, are strongly expressing a desire to work (Department of Health, 2001). With the employment level at less than 10% for this particular group of disabled people, this presents a considerable challenge. There is a widespread view that the great majority of people with learning difficulties are not able to engage in paid work and would be vulnerable to exploitation if they did. The minority who do work, however, do so in a broad range of settings, with widely varying levels of ability, so competence would not seem to be the major issue. In addition, paid work is seen as a highly valued occupation; it provides employees with more money than welfare benefit claimants, and more income means more choice in the market for goods and services and therefore increases the control of their lives.

In order to explore further the position of people with learning difficulties in relation to the employment market, we need to look at the legislation, policy and systems in place to facilitate people with learning difficulties and disabled people more generally into jobs. But what about social work and social workers? What part might social workers play in these policies and systems? What are the traditions of social work that might encourage social workers to engage with the system?

THE DEVELOPMENT OF SOCIAL WORK VISIONS

In reflecting upon the role of social work I have gone back over the development of my understanding of the social work role in the time that I have been involved with social work practice. I started as an unqualified social worker in the early 1970s. I was naïve and inexperienced, but at least had some understanding of social injustice and the politics that created it, so it did not take much to recognise that the people I worked with were invariably the poor, marginalised and dispossessed. I also found many of the people that I was asked to visit to be friendless and seen as unacceptable within their families and local communities. In my lowly position I was given little training or supervision in anything apart from correct procedures, so had little idea what to do apart from offer what I have come to term unconditional positive regard and probably create a great deal of dependency!

As a social work undergraduate in the mid-seventies, and in the period immediately after qualifying as a social worker, I had begun to recognise the role of community development in identifying the needs of communities. I had learnt that individual needs could, in some cases, be met better through the development and support of informal networks that were non-stigmatising, unlike the newly emergent Social Services Departments. In practice, however, Social Services Departments continued their focus on individuals, largely assessed and processed with little regard to their strengths or the strengths of the families or communities within which they lived.

From the mid-80s up until now we have, in social work, recognised the *specific* ways in which people who receive health and social care services experience collective marginalisation, discrimination and oppression. As a result of this recognition we have developed models of understanding and action (Taylor and Baldwin, 1991) such as Anti- Racism (Dominelli, 1988; Ahmad, 1990), Anti-Discriminatory Practice (Thompson, 1993), and empowerment (Dalrymple & Burke, 1995; Braye & Preston-Shoot, 1995), built upon theoretical models such as the social model of disability (Oliver, 1996) and normalisation (Oliver & Barnes, 1998). What we are increasingly recognising, as we require social work students on placement to demonstrate evidence of their practice within these models and theoretical frameworks, is that empowerment in a context of low resources, and continuing individual and institutional discrimination in social welfare organisations, is at least a tall order, if not actually an exercise in setting students up to fail.

More recently, from the early 1990s, we have begun to recognise that involvement by people who use social work services (service users) is one of the keys to ensuring that their needs are met. Learning about service user-focused or service user-led assessment and needs-led assessment has transformed the way we think, as social workers, about the power relationships involved in decision-making in the allocation of scarce resources. Service users are also involved in researching potential new service initiatives that may affect their life chances. They are also becoming more involved in the evaluation of programmes, training staff, and planning, managing, teaching and assessing on social work degree programs (Sadd & Baldwin, 2005).

So, what we have seen in social work is a progression from recognising exclusion, working on inclusion within local communities, understanding discrimination and oppression and the limits to empowering practice within statutory organisations, and latterly starting to test out the extent to which service users can be more involved in decisions that affect their lives. But to what extent are social workers, working with people with learning difficulties, engaging with policy mechanisms within their organisations and networks, to make these values a reality in their practice?

POLICY DEVELOPMENTS IN THE UK

There are different kinds of policy and legislation that I want to focus upon. Some of the policy and legislation is facilitative–designed to ensure that policy objectives are met. There is also protective legislation, such as the Disability Discrimination Acts, which is designed to ensure that barriers to policy implementation are broken down.

As indicated above, the Social Exclusion Unit within the New Labour Government has expressed a belief that it is access to work that is the best route to social inclusion for groups such as disabled people. In addition, the Cabinet Office has expressly argued the case for paid employment as the key to improving disabled people's life chances (Cabinet Office, 2005). So what are the policy devices that have been developed to put this policy into practice? I want to look at how systems are being developed in the UK to enable disabled people generally to get into work–and to what extent they include people with learning difficulties.

White Paper–Valuing People: A New Strategy for Learning Disability in the 21st Century (2001)

This is a remarkable policy document, published in March 2001 and driven to a substantial degree by the interests of people with learning difficulties. A process of inclusion was built into the construction of the policy document and it is not surprising, therefore, that it has an empowering ethos at its heart. The policy document has been written in accessible format and geared primarily towards people with learning difficulties. There are clear messages for commissioners of services and service providers, but the focus is first and foremost on informing the service user group themselves, of what the policy intentions are.

As a white paper, *Valuing People* provides the policy framework for this area. First I will explore the details relating to employment in this policy document before picking out some of the key areas for further analysis.

"The government believes that employment is an important route to social inclusion and that all those that wish to work should have the opportunity and support to do so" (Department of Health, 2001: 84). This statement is an unequivocal declaration that people with learning difficulties are not to be left out of the government policy that argues work as the key to social inclusion. The White Paper acknowledges the problem of low employment for people with learning difficulties (less than 10%), and that it may not be a "realistic option for all," but real jobs and wages are a "major aspiration for many" (Department of Health, 2001: 84).

The White Paper argues that social exclusion for people with learning difficulties has been as a result of a number of disabling factors. Low expectations from local authority staff and others who are there to provide support to people is a clear indication that services provide a disabling environment for people with learning difficulties. Low expectations inevitably lead to poor training and support for people with learning difficulties. The White Paper also notes that there is poor interaction between the benefits system and employment, and that these create disincentives. One of the government schemes to assist the movement of disabled people into employment–Supported Employment (sheltered work environments)–is argued as a poor route to mainstream employment for people with learning difficulties (Department of Health, 2001).

Other Policies to Assist Disabled People into the Labor Market

There are then a range of key areas of policy activity by government to meet the overall aim of increasing the numbers of people with learning difficulties in work. These include the New Labour policy instrument of targets for increasing numbers of people with learning difficulties in work. There is an initiative known as the Workstep program which is, in effect, sheltered workshops, not paid employment, but with an emphasis on transition for those who can enter the job market. A new DoH/ DWP scoping study to look at links between supported employment and day services was proposed in the White Paper. Again, the intention here is to see how more traditional approaches, such as day services, could facilitate the transition into the job market. The New Deal for Disabled People is part of a broader government initiative to facilitate the inclusion of people who are seen as priorities. One of the practical corollaries of this policy initiative is to ensure that Job Brokers have the skills to work with people with learning difficulties, following their success with other groups such as lone parents (Department of Health, 2001).

Disability Living Allowance is part of the welfare benefit system designed to support disabled people, but it does create disincentives for some to move into work. The White Paper announced steps to remove those disincentives and actually provide motivation within the benefits system for people to move into paid employment (Department of Health, 2001).

Learning Disability Partnership Boards were one of the practical initiatives that have come from the White Paper. They are designed to be inclusive local policy development mechanisms that will involve people with learning difficulties in decision-making on the development of a broad range of local services and initiatives. As part of their brief, Partnership Boards are required to develop local employment strategies. Local authorities are recognised as an important potential source of employment for disabled people and are, through the White Paper, encouraged to develop better employment prospects for people with learning difficulties. This is backed by the disability rights legislation (see p. 103 for more detail) that includes a duty on public bodies to promote disability equality. To support this legislation the government has also set targets for employment of disabled people (which at least in principle would include people with learning difficulties) (Department of Health, 2001).

There are, in addition to the above policy proposals, a number of other initiatives. These include Disabled Persons' Tax credits that reduce disincentives to work and enable the process of transition from benefits to (often low-paid) work. There have been improvements to the Incapacity Benefit that will assist people as they move into the world of work with its inevitable uncertainties and false starts. People will now be entitled to re-qualification if they leave work, whereas before, their entitlement was terminated. The Independent Living Fund, another benefit to assist those meeting eligibility criteria relating to chronic illness and disability, is also being tweaked to ensure greater incentives in the transition to paid employment. There is to be a higher earnings disregard for people in work, and new rules allow disabled people to use this benefit alongside of Direct Payments (see below), for example, employment of a support worker to facilitate someone's move into employment. It is also the case that the minimum wage as a universalist policy initiative has improved the prospects for disabled people to earn a living wage, rather than pocket money from therapeutic employment (Department of Health, 2001).

Direct Payments

This initiative takes access to some financial resources for disabled people away from the benefit system and was introduced by the Conservative government through the Community Care (Direct Payments) Act in 1997. Direct Payments (DP) are cash payments to people who are eligible for Social Services Department adult care services, to enable them to purchase their own support. Such support may come from local authority or LA commissioned services but would not necessarily do so. It allows disabled people the freedom to spend the money in a way that provides their solution to a perceived problem, rather than being tied to more traditional and general service provisions.

Initially Direct Payments were limited to people aged 18-65, and were denied to older people and people with learning difficulties. As a result of heavy lobbying, direct payments were extended to these groups of potential beneficiaries. This lobbying included the presentation of research carried out by people with learning difficulties that proved they COULD manage direct payments with assistance.

Direct payments can be seen as one of the most empowering initiatives of broader community care policy, inasmuch as they appear to give people who have been dependent upon traditional services an opportunity to have a voice in the kind and blend of resources that might be made available to meet their assessed needs. What are the benefits and barriers to this new form of payment? Glasby and Littlechild (2002) who have talked with people in receipt of direct payments argue the benefits to be, firstly, more responsive services in which service users can exercise more choice and control. This in turn has improved their morale and well-being, a finding that fits convincingly with the theory of human need argued by Doyal and Gough (1991) in which autonomy is one of the universal prerequisites for the meeting of need. Direct Payments provide this degree of autonomy and the result is an increase in well-being as the Doyal/Gough model would predict (Glasby & Littlechild, 2002). Direct Payments are also argued as leading to more creative use of resources. Rather than reliance on a one-size-fits-all approach of more traditional services, direct payments free up service users and their careers to think laterally about individualised approaches to meeting their care needs. Glasby and Littlechild (2002) also found that there was a reduced cost or, at the least, better value for money for services purchased with direct payments.

Glasby and Littlechild (2002) do note barriers to these benefits, however. The principle barrier concerns the related issues of competence and consent. According to the regulations attached to the legislation, those in receipt of a direct payment must be willing and able to receive a Direct Payment. What Glasby and Littlechild (2002) quoted was the disabling assumptions from social workers about who is competent and, therefore, able to give consent (Dawson, 2000).

A failure to provide accessible information to people with learning difficulties plus the complexity of the bureaucratic system has also proved to be a barrier. The latter point, interestingly, given the focus in this article about the practice of social workers, is that the systems of assessment and monitoring find social workers displaying little motivation or commitment. There is also evidence that organisations are using unofficial rationing systems to deny access to Direct Payments for people likely to incur the more costly support services. There is also evidence from my own research of the use of other blanket criteria to deny access to Direct Payments for rationing purposes. In one authority I have investigated there is a rule that nobody is allowed to apply for a Direct Payment until they are over 18, a rule which is actually *ultra vires*.

I want, now, to look at these barriers, and how they are being dealt with, in a little more detail as there would appear to be evidence of organisations and the individuals within them bending the rules, or at the least applying them rigidly, in order to deny people with learning difficulties access to resources that could be utilised in their quest to enter the labour market. This would seem to be at least prima facie evidence of professionals using their discretion, with or without organisational connivance, to undermine the intentions of the broader policy framework, and, therefore, acting as Street Level Bureaucrats in the way described by Lipsky (1980).

"Consent" has been re-categorised by subsequent Department of Health guidance (Department of Health, 2004) as firstly an agreement and an indication of preference, rather than its prior more legalistic conceptualisation. The guidance also describes consent as a process rather than an event of assessment. This is in recognition that many disabled people, perhaps especially those with learning difficulties, can be enabled to understand complex ideas such as consent over time. There is evidence, for instance (Baldwin, 1997), of people with learning difficulties being given an opportunity to learn what a choice is and how to make one, in a mutually supportive environment.

There is some recognition, in recent guidance, that the bureaucracy is necessarily legalistic and that legal contracts are required. The fact that many applicants will require advocates to assist in this legal process should not be used as evidence that individuals are incompetent (Department of Health, 2004). Everyone utilises the professional knowledge and skills of lawyers for some transactions. Outside of disabling attitudes, it is hard to explain why some are deemed incompetent if they are unable to engage with particular legal processes without such assistance. My research has indicated that resistance by some social workers to the bureaucracy is on the grounds of its complexity. Specialist workers in the Direct Payment field believe that the bureaucracy is perceived to be more complex than it actually is.

The message from guidance is that "support available is key" (Department of Health, 2004: 5) to success. The Department of Health has reframed this aspect of the Direct Payment initiative so that support is not viewed as "contrary to independent living but a crucial component of it" (Department of Health, 2004: 5). Support is seen as necessary for people with learning difficulties to manage employment issues, budgets, etc. The types of support available are manifold and include local authority dedicated workers, staff from independent support organisations, Circles of Support, user controlled Independent Living Trusts and legal structures. An additional and pertinent source of support is self-advocacy or peer support from other more experienced people with learning difficulties. Leadership, which is a new venture in recognising, validating and building upon such expertise, is ensuring there are "champions at all levels" (Department of Health, 2004: 12), including people with learning difficulties. Support from such leaders is seen as not only being more effective in that it will often be provided by people who have direct experience of ways of working through bureaucratic procedures, but it is also seen as crucial for morale and to ensure access to information (Department of Health, 2004).

To work through these barriers, despite the new guidance from the Department of Health, will require a change of ethos in Social Services Departments. There is evidence that the attitudes and the approach of local authority and staff have greatly influenced take-up of Direct Payments (Bewley & McCulloch, 2002). Examples from this particular piece of research included social workers and first-line managers expressing their own personal views that people with learning difficulties should not have access to Direct Payments, regardless of rules. In addition there is a fear of resource implications should there be an increased take-up of Direct Payments, fear of increased demands from Support Agencies, and concerns that local authority services are set up for different purposes (Bewley & McCulloch, 2002). Hence the argument that the changes required are in attitude and behaviour rather than resources. Indeed, as with mental health services in the UK, there is also a suggestion that a new type of worker is required, one who understands the requirements of service user-focused and needs-led assessment, and who can act as a champion for service users.

As far as accessibility of information is concerned, it is argued that people with learning difficulties do not need *different* information as is claimed–but *accessible* information. There is a persuasive argument that more accessible information provision by local authorities about services available would assist all services users and not just those with particular communication problems.

Direct Payments are also criticised for other factors that are of relevance to their usage as a potential tool for the transition for people with learning difficulties into the labour market. Jenny Morris (2005), for instance, criticises Direct Payments for a focus on individual consumerism, rather than providing a recognition of the collective experience of disability and making a more generalist provision for breaking down barriers for disabled people getting access to social goods such as employment. She also argues that the limitations on budgets for Direct Payments effectively push down wages for careers employed with Direct Payments by disabled people to provide them with essential support (Morris, 2005).

Her argument about choice as a cornerstone of government policy is that choice needs to come with control and human rights for service users if it is to have any meaning. And if it is a policy with value for the government, and it requires more resources to make it work, then money should be provided rather than undermining the value of the policy by withholding adequate resources. Jenny Morris argues her case for linking choice, rights, autonomy, participation and contribution–within arguments on citizenship–most persuasively. If governments are serious about disabled people being socially included as equal citizens, then their choices must come as a right, must be made as autonomous actors who can both participate in and contribute to the common good as fellow citizens.

Access to Work Programme

The Access to Work Programme (Job Centre Plus Website) is designed for people who meet the statutory definition of a "disabled person" and need extra practical help to access employment and hold down a job. Job Centre Plus, the organisation that implements the programme, offers advice on solutions in three areas:

- physical and environmental aids and adaptations
- human support on the job or getting to work–including job coaches
- fares to and from work

Research indicates that nine out of 10 people on the scheme were already in work when it started. It is, as a scheme, more geared to retention of current workers than recruitment of new disabled employees, so would not, at present, seem to be of much use for the 90% of people with learning difficulties who are out of work. In the future, however, it may provide a blueprint for the kind of assistance that new recruits to the labour market might draw upon. It is used currently for communication support for disabled people at interview, to employ support workers, which could include specialist coaching for people with learning difficulties, as well as special equipment an individual requires such as adaptations to working environments not covered under employer liability from the Disability Discrimination legislation (as follows), and travel costs.

There is no evaluation of this scheme as yet. My research interviews with professionals in the field found them to be sceptical, especially in relation to people with learning difficulties, for whom access is non-existent at present.

Supported Employment Services (Workstep)

This scheme which has been re-branded as Workstep in recent years provides sheltered working schemes rather than mainstream employment. Evidence indicates that there is poor transition from sheltered work schemes into the mainstream job market. At the 16-years-of-age transition period young people with learning difficulties tend to go into college or sheltered employment schemes, so miss this crucial window of opportunity for transition into paid employment.

RESEARCH ON DISABLED PEOPLE'S ACCESS TO EMPLOYMENT

It is worth looking at a major literature review of access to work by disabled people to see what some of the barriers to work are for disabled people in general. The additional barrier of a learning difficulty would seem to suggest that these barriers are likely to be of equal force if not worse for people with learning difficulties.

The research reviewed in this publication found that disabled applicants for jobs have less than an equal chance of being considered for a job they have applied for; 28% of disabled respondents said discrimination made it harder for them to access and then retain work and 16% said they had experienced discrimination at work. Most public bodies indicated that they knew about employment of disabled people and available schemes for support, but this was not the case for people with learning difficulties (Hirst, Thornton, Dearey, & Maynard Campbell, 2004).

DISABILITY DISCRIMINATION LEGISLATION AND THE DISABILITY RIGHTS COMMISSION

As some of the above evidence suggests that people with learning difficulties experience discrimination getting access to resources to support them into the labour market, as well as in accessing paid employment, I need to look at the legislation on the statute book to outlaw discrimination against disabled people.

The Disability Discrimination Act of 1995 made it unlawful to discriminate against a disabled person and noted this specifically in relation to employee status. The Act also introduced the concept of "reasonable adjustment" in which employers are required under law to make such adjustments in working procedures, practices and environments to accommodate disabled people.

The Disability Discrimination Act of 2005 amended the earlier legislation, setting up the statutory Disability Rights Commission to oversee compliance with the legislation. It also introduced a duty on all public bodies to "promote disability equality." Specifically this places a duty on public bodies such as local authorities to produce "disability equality schemes" in partnership with other local bodies–designed to progress recruitment, retention and career development of disabled people. These schemes should include people with learning difficulties as they are designated as disabled people under the original legislation.

In principle at least, this recent legislation ought to provide the statutory framework to ensure rights of access to social goods such as employment in much the same way that Jenny Morris (2005) suggested.

INDEPENDENCE, WELL-BEING AND CHOICE– GREEN PAPER (2005)

This consultation document, produced by the Department of Health and subtitled "Our Vision for the Future of Social Care for Adults in England," has some interesting and important policy aims that fit with some of the arguments that I have explored in this article so far. They have direct and indirect implications for people with learning difficulties and the labour market.

The focus of the consultation document is "independence through choice"–again that New Labour word "choice" being at the centre of the policy initiative. The Green paper makes links with social inclusion, declaring that all organisations involved with "adults," by which they mean those people who are eligible for services under the community care legislation, have a responsibility to ensure that these groups, which would include people with learning difficulties, are socially included. Given the Social Exclusion Unit's focus on work as the key method of ensuring inclusion, it is not surprising that there is mention of work as a part of the policy intention. The key presented here is prevention, with a requirement for organisations to streamline assessment of entitlement to services. Where this is related to work, the emphasis is on improving communications and procedures between local authorities and the central government body responsible for employment–the Department of Work and Pensions. In relation to this and other promises of choice for eligible adults, the Green Paper requires local authorities to meet targets for increased take-up of Direct Payments. A new initiative is Individual Budgets, which are intended to provide individual resources for service users who may not wish, or be able, to make use of Direct Payments. This would seem to deal with one of the barriers around competence relating to Direct Payments noted above, although the time scale is set between publication and 2012, leaving many people with learning difficulties at transition stages where they might gain paid employment with that kind of support, at the mercy of current disabling service provision.

With the latter proviso, this would seem to be a consultation document that supports other initiatives mentioned.

CONCLUSIONS

There remains some concern about the nature of employment for people with learning difficulties in the labour market, and whether exploitation could be an inhibiting factor. But, in the absence of any firm evidence of this one way or the other, and accepting that many people with learning difficulties want to gain paid employment, it useful to evaluate the effectiveness of the policy frameworks (legislative, organisational, and practice) in place to facilitate this process. This article has presented some of the necessary evidence for this evaluation. I want to end by summarising this and concluding with what we know and what still needs to be explored and, more tellingly, what needs to be done to ensure the maximum take-up of realistic paid work by people with learning difficulties so that they can move from welfare to work.

Government policy about employment and social inclusion could not be clearer. I have quoted above the expectations of government that also suggest there will be a broad range of measures and resources put in place to ensure that disabled people are given opportunities for employment. As we have seen, the legislation provides a framework for disability rights, which include the right to fair treatment in accessing employment and being employed. This legislation *should* include people with learning difficulties as they are one of the groups covered by the legislation. Evaluation-wise, this is a salient point. Organisation and practice should include people with learning difficulties. But how successfully are people with learning difficulties being included? There are problems with funding, but the greater problem seems to be with the required change in ethos, attitudes and behaviour of all involved in working with people with learning difficulties.

Social workers, in collaboration with others–personal advisers, transitions workers, job brokers, job coaches, and employers–have the policy framework and some financial levers to facilitate people with learning difficulties into work. It would seem that, for people with learning difficulties, employment as an aspect of empowering practice is not on some of the key practitioners' agenda. We have evidence of disabling attitudes only gradually changing, and service-driven responses rather than imaginative planning with people for their futures.

In order to be clear about these apparent barriers, there needs to be further research into what the nature of the threats to this form of empowering practice are, and why it is that organisations are not utilising the available policy, legal frameworks, and the financial resources for enabling people with learning difficulties to enter the labour market.

Addressing what needs to happen can be explored by returning to the unfolding value base for social work that I outlined at the start of this article. In doing so we can note the distance that is still to be travelled by organisations and practitioners before this particular marginalised group receives fair treatment within values-based organisation and practice. The individualism within which so much social work practice operates ignores the collective marginalisation that people with learning difficulties experience. Individual blocks to employment are then easy to erect and utilise as excuses for what are actually generalised disabling attitudes and practices. The fact that only 10% of people with learning difficulties are in paid employment would suggest that there is a powerful collective resistance to their employment. Although not all people with learning difficulties could hold down paid work, competence would not seem to be the major factor, as many people are in valued employment in a broad range of settings.

Recognition of this collective experience of marginalisation, plus a more focused approach to the expressed needs and wishes of individuals, the case is more likely to result in social workers helping people with learning difficulties meet their aspirations. It is the case, as has been noted in the White Paper–Valuing People–and the research into attitudes and practices recorded above, that it is these attitudes that are the key stumbling block to policy implementation. Disabling attitudes are not what we might expect from social workers in the 21st century, so it is to be hoped that the anti-discrimination legislation (Disability Discrimination Acts of 1995 and 2005) and the codes of practice for social workers (General Social Care Council, 2002) which outlaw such attitudes and, indeed, require social workers to promote disability equality, will swiftly consign disabling attitudes to the dustbin of history. Social workers, working in partnership with people with learning difficulties and other allies, can then start to recognise and deal with some of the other barriers to employment that exist within the labour market.

REFERENCES

Ahmad, B. (1990). *Black Perspectives in Social Work*. Birmingham: Venture Press.

Baldwin, M. (1997). Day care on the move: Learning from a participative action research project at a day centre for people with learning difficulties. *British Journal of Social Work, 27*(6), 951-958.

Bewley, C., & McCulloch, L. (2002). *Helping Ourselves: Direct Payments and the Development of Peer Support*. London: Values into Action.

Braye, S., & Preston-Shoot, M. (1995). *Empowering Practice in Social Care*. Buckingham: Open University Press.

Cabinet Office (2005). *Improving the Life Chances of Disabled People*. London: Strategy Unit/Cabinet Office.

Clegg, D. (2005). A rootless Third Way: A continental European perspective on New Labour's welfare state, re-visited. In M. Powell, L. Bauld, & K. Clarke (Eds.), *Social Policy Review 17: Analysis and Debate in Social Policy, 2005*. Bristol: The Policy Press, pp. 233-253.

Dalrymple, J., & Burke, B. (1995). *Anti-Oppressive Practice: Social Care and the Law*. Buckingham: Open University Press.

Dawson, C. (2000). Independent successes: Implementing direct payments. Cited in J. Glasby & R. Littlechild, *Social Work and Direct Payments*. Bristol: The Policy Press.

Department of Health (2001). *Valuing People: A New Strategy for Learning Disability for the 21st Century. A White Paper*. London: HMSO.

Department of Health (2004). *Direct Choices: What Councils Need to Make Direct Payments Happen for People with Learning Disabilities*. London: HMSO.

Department of Health (2005). *Independence, Well-Being and Choice–Green Paper*. London: HMSO.

Dominelli, L. (1988). *Anti-Racist Social Work: A Challenge for White Practitioners and Educators*. Basingstoke: Macmillan.

Doyal, L., & Gough, I. (1991). *A Theory of Human Need*. Basingstoke: Macmillan.

General Social Care Council (2002). *Codes of Practice for Social Care Workers and Employers*. London: General Social Care Council.

Glasby, J., & Littlechild, R. (2002). *Social Work and Direct Payments*. Bristol: The Policy Press.

Hirst, M., Thornton, P., Dearey, M., & Maynard Campbell, S. (2004). *The Employment of Disabled People in the Public Sector: A Review of Data and Literature*. London: Disability Rights Commission.

Job Centre Plus Website. *http://www.jobcentreplus.gov.uk/cms.asp?Page=/Home/Customers/HelpForDisabledPeople/AccesstoWork*.

Levitas, R. (1998). *The Inclusive Society*. Basingstoke: Macmillan.

Lipsky, M. (1980). *Street Level Bureaucrats: Dilemmas of the Individual in Public Services*. New York: Russell Sage Foundation.

Morris, J. (2005). *Independent Living: The Role of Evidence and Ideology in the Development of Government Policy*. Paper presented to the conference Cash and Care: Understanding the Evidence Base for Policy and Practice, April 12 &13, 2005, University of York (Sally Baldwin Memorial Conference).

Office of the Deputy Prime Minister (2003). *Tackling Social Exclusion: Achievements, Lessons Learnt and the Way Forward*. London: Office of the Deputy Prime Minister and the Social Exclusion Unit.

Oliver, M. (1996). *Understanding Disability: From Theory to Practice*. Basingstoke: Macmillan.

Oliver, M., & Barnes, C. (1998). *Disabled People and Social Policy: From Exclusion to Inclusion*. Harlow: Longman.

Powell, M., Bauld, L., & Clarke, K. (Eds) (2005). *Social Policy Review 17: Analysis and Debate in Social Policy, 2005*. Bristol: The Policy Press.

Sadd, J., & Baldwin, M. (2006, forthcoming). Allies with attitude! Service users, academics and social service agency staff learning how to share power in running social work education programmes. *Social Work Education, 24*(4).

Taylor, P., & Baldwin, M. (1991). Travelling hopefully: Anti-racist practice and practice learning opportunities. *Social Work Education, 10* (3): 5-32.

Thompson, N. (1993). *Anti-Discriminatory Practice*. Basingstoke: Macmillan.

Workfare Oz-Style:
Welfare Reform and Social Work
in Australia

Catherine McDonald
Lesley Chenoweth

SUMMARY. Traditional approaches to the promotion of welfare have disappeared in Australia, replaced by a new institutional order represented by welfare-cum-workfare. This has impacted on social work–both as a collective entity and as a set of practices. This paper maps the shift to workfare in Australia and examines its impacts on and implications for social work. We briefly discuss the Australian model of social protection, illustrating our own brand of "exceptionalism," and lay out what we have termed "Workfare Oz-style." Drawing upon neo-institutional theory, we review and analyze two key contexts where "Workfare Oz-style" is operationalized–the Job Network and Centrelink. Some tentative conclusions are given and the dimensions of a research agenda, which will put any emerging propositions to empirical test, are proposed. *[Article copies available for a fee from The Haworth Document Delivery Service: 1-800-HAWORTH. E-mail address: <docdelivery@haworthpress.com> Website: <http://www. HaworthPress.com> © 2006 by The Haworth Press, Inc. All rights reserved.]*

Catherine McDonald, PhD, is Senior Lecturer, School of Social Work and Applied Human Sciences, The University of Queensland, Brisbane 2LD4072, Australia. Lesley Chenoweth, PhD, is Professor, Social Work, Logan Campus, University Drive, Griffith University, MEADOWBROOK QLD 4131, Australia.

[Haworth co-indexing entry note]: "Workfare Oz-Style: Welfare Reform and Social Work in Australia." McDonald, Catherine, and Lesley Chenoweth. Co-published simultaneously in *Journal of Policy Practice* (The Haworth Press, Inc.) Vol. 5, No. 2/3, 2006, pp. 109-128; and: *International Perspectives on Welfare to Work Policy* (ed: Richard Hoefer, and James Midgley) The Haworth Press, Inc., 2006, pp. 109-128. Single or multiple copies of this article are available for a fee from The Haworth Document Delivery Service [1-800- HAWORTH, 9:00 a.m. - 5:00 p.m. (EST). E-mail address: docdelivery@haworthpress.com].

Available online at http://www.haworthpress.com/web/JPP
© 2006 by The Haworth Press, Inc. All rights reserved.
doi:10.1300/J508v05n02_08

KEYWORDS. Social work, welfare, welfare reform, social policy, Australian social work

INTRODUCTION

In a recent conversation with the two most senior social workers in Australia's Federal (Commonwealth) bureaucracy, one of them commented that Australian social workers are like the frogs in that proverbial pot of hot water, except that the water is well and truly boiling and has been for some time. What was interesting about this comment was its metaphorical acknowledgment that Australian social workers–even those at the forefront of the changes we call "workfare"–are less than fully aware of what is happening, and what has already happened to them.

This lack of awareness is salient and a function of several factors–both structural and deliberative. First, the way the welfare regime is structured in Australia positions social workers in such diverse locations that there is little commonality of experience. Awareness of institutional change is, at best, muted and partial. Second, and perhaps more importantly, there has been no "big bang" restructuring the universe of welfare such as the U.S. Personal Responsibility and Work Opportunity Reconciliation Act, 1996. Rather, the policy trajectory and programmatic responses to the ideas of workfare have been incremental, bipartisan, and in many instances, slipped in under the guise of public sector reform.

In reality, welfare reform associated with contemporary workfare began in Australia as early as the second half of the 1980s with what was known as the Social Security Review (Cass, 1986). Following OECD prescriptions, reform of income security in tandem with the introduction of active labor market programs were subsequently developed by the (supposedly) left-of-center Labor government culminating in 1994 with the *Working Nation* program (Keating, 1994; Finn, 1999). The long lead up to contemporary workfare initiatives has resulted in a situation in which the resultant programs are not considered in any way remarkable, and are positioned by government in public discourse as a natural consequence of social and economic developments. This, we suggest, indicates that the transition to Workfare Oz-style represents successful institutional transformation (Phillips, Lawrence, & Hardy, 2004).

Further, the overt ideologies of workfare are entirely congruent with a modal (even iconic) Australian identity of the working man or "battler" (Turner, 1995), predicated on blue collar and lower white collar (male) labor force participation. In such a context it is entirely possible that few

Australians appreciate the implications of the type and degree of institutional transformation wrought by "Workfare Oz-style," not least of which to the traditional Aussie battler in a post-industrial economy. Yet this transformation is the bottom-line, reflecting a reconfiguration of what was known locally as the "Australian Way" (Smyth & Cass, 1998). Paralleling developments noted by commentators about other modern welfare regimes (Gilbert, 2002; Glennerster, 1999), Workfare Oz-style actually represents a fundamental refashioning of the regime choices Australia made in the early part of the 20th Century.

This paper focuses on social work in particular, proposing a preliminary premise that social work was/is a key expression of modernity represented in traditional Keynesian-inspired approaches to 20th Century welfare. While being aware of the contested nature of the field (see Castles, 1983) we also advance a second premise that the traditional approaches to the promotion of welfare have gone. A new institutional order represented by welfare-cum-workfare is in place (Jessop, 2002) which, logically, impacts on social work–both as a collective entity and as a set of practices.

To map what has happened and what is likely to happen in the near future to Australian social work, we first briefly discuss the Australian model of social protection, illustrating our own brand of "exceptionalism" (except that New Zealand did it too). We do this to underscore the dimensions of institutional transformation in the march to Workfare Oz-style. Second, we set the scene for appreciating the specific local operations of workfare and the implications for social work, discussing Australian federalism, "Workfare Oz-style" and Australian social work. Third, we offer two key contexts where "Workfare Oz-style" is being operationalized–the Job Network and Centrelink. Finally, we pose some tentative conclusions, and spell out the dimensions of a research agenda which will put any emerging propositions to an empirical test.

THE AUSTRALIAN CONTEXT

The Australian Way

Reflecting an historic compromise between labor and capital, the mature Australian welfare regime developed into an institutional order, which upheld citizenship rights–although primarily as industrial rights of working men (Wearing, 1994). In the interests of protecting the viability of its industrializing economy, Australia developed a comprehensive system of tariff protection and a legislatively protected centralized wage fixing system in the first half of the 20th century. In what was known as the "wage earners' welfare state," wage fixing became the primary mode of institutional redistribution (Castles, 1983). This crucial process was complemented by legislated occupational entitlements (sick leave, recreation leave, and eventually superannuation). Australian (male) wages were kept artificially high, a system which both encouraged and allowed families to meet their own needs, embedding a deep, though false, sense of self-reliance. Other health, education and social services developed incrementally, largely in response to differentiated interest mobilization.

As the 20th century progressed, a highly targeted and selective social protection scheme, funded through Commonwealth general tax revenue, was established for dependent populations falling outside of the labor market. These were groups which the wage earners' welfare state largely ignored–the aged, the disabled, orphans, widows, single supporting mothers, and the unemployed. In a context where the states have limited tax powers, health, education, and welfare were also funded primarily by the Commonwealth government through general *untied* grants to the states, delivered through a complex mixed economy of welfare. Wage fixing aside, the overall orientation of the Australian welfare state was nevertheless fairly reluctant, patchy, parsimonious and in the case of income security, stigmatizing.

During the early 1970s, this essentially piecemeal approach was abruptly overhauled, and a short period of extensive welfare state building began. Through a variety of measures the selectivity of the Australian system was partially, yet significantly reversed as the Australian Government reconstructed itself as the primary vehicle for the carriage of *social,* not just industrial rights. Substantial efforts were made to overhaul the income security system, slightly decreasing its selectivity and opening it up to previously excluded groups such as single mothers. This was an aberrant period in Australian welfare history, but it was highly influential in that it swung the pendulum away from being a welfare laggard to a more comprehensive liberal welfare state with some clear social democratic tendencies, for example, universal health care.

Unfortunately, this expansionary social democratically-informed period coincided with global economic processes which fundamentally rewrote the historic compromise and firmly squashed any tendencies towards social democratic ideals.

The Path to "Workfare Oz-Style"

The 1970s brief social democratic turn in the Australian welfare state was, during the last two decades of the 20th century, steadily overturned. More importantly, economic globalization and the associated rise and eventual dominance of neoclassical economics and neo-liberal politics played a key role in destabilizing and eventually completely fragmenting the long-standing Australian compromise between capital and labor. The central plank of the Australian system, centralized wage fixing, was steadily dismantled rendering the wage earners' welfare state an historical artifact. Further, the removal of the tariff walls opened up the Australian economy to that complex of global economic forces that, as happened in other industrialized nations, reconfigured industry and the domestic labor market.

In addition, macroeconomic policy prioritized the reduction of inflation over employment generation, and as a consequence, unemployment and underemployment grew rapidly. Not surprisingly, the traditional reliance on full-time life-long employment (upon which the original model was predicated) became redundant. Further, sustained Commonwealth government fixation with reducing budget deficits heralded an unrelenting fiscal squeeze and associated widespread cuts in funding for social services. Australian governments on both sides of politics became increasingly disengaged from direct service delivery and more and more services were devolved to the other sectors, including the informal sector. As such, the long-standing reliance on a mixed economy of welfare was reinforced. Further, vigorous application of the nostrums of New Public Management (Osborne & Gaebler, 1992; Peters, 1996) ensured that state control of the mixed economy of welfare through such mechanisms as the contract, audit, risk and the quality agenda escalated.

At the same time and in keeping with the OECD recommendations, Australian income security policy began to undo any pretence of social citizenship rights, and fractured the dependent population back into the categories of deserving and undeserving poor. Unlike the USA with its focus on welfare mothers, the primary target to date has been the long-term unemployed who have, since 1997, been drawn into a coercive workfare program emphasizing claimant obligations as opposed to rights.

As yet, the Australian system has not managed to embroil state governments, and significant areas of service delivery where social workers are most often engaged remain relatively unaffected by the rationalities of workfare. However, more recent Federal government policy initiatives seek to extend the workfare regime to people with disabilities and single supporting parents, which will roll out over the next three years. In summary, the combination of reversing commitment to redistribution via wage deregulation, the ongoing commitment to containing inflation at the expense of employment, the reshaping of the labor market, the fiscal parsimony, and the linking of income security with employment policy have all lead to the emergence of an understated, barely acknowledged and poorly understood workfare regime in Australia.

THE IMPLICATIONS OF FEDERALISM

Like the USA, Australia is a federated political system. The Australian states provide the bulk of social services (child welfare, health, disability services, education, and public housing). While the Commonwealth has steadily attempted to permeate state social policies and programs with its own policy prescriptions, its capacity to do so is structurally limited by the Australian constitution. As indicated, state grants are, for the most part, untied. So despite the existence of significant vertical-fiscal imbalance whereby the Commonwealth has the taxing powers and the states the spending responsibilities, the Commonwealth cannot, as yet, directly shape state-provided welfare. Rather it is forced to influence by negotiating rolling funding "agreements" on a state-by-state and field-specific basis. Accordingly, the Australian states have traditionally acted as a moderating force in Commonwealth social policy agendas.

In welfare reform, there is little evidence as yet at the state level that social services have been drawn in. That said, the states are concerned about the impact on their own patterns of expenditure. Recent swings in the constantly moving pendulum of federalism indicate that the Commonwealth will launch an offensive on states' autonomy (signaled in health, education and well underway in industrial relations). Recently, it gained control of the upper House of Parliament (the Senate). Now, the Coalition controls both Houses, making the conditions ripe for widespread structural change. Welfare reform has been identified as a primary policy target for such changes and as of July 1, 2006, supporting mothers and people with disabilities will be drawn into the reform agenda along with the unemployed.

While there have been constitutional impediments to a complete Commonwealth dominance of social policy agendas, each of the states have accepted and introduced the principles of New Public Management into their social welfare service delivery. As a consequence, market and consumer orientations attendant to such developments have seriously influenced social services at the point of delivery. While state-based social services are not as yet formally implicated directly in Workfare Oz-style, the rationality or institutional logic of marketized and corporatized service delivery has swept virtually every sector of Australian social services. This, we suggest, indicates that the ground-work has already been done, and when Commonwealth-state relations change, the spread of workfare-like principles and practices will not meet much resistance across state welfare sectors.

Social Work in Australia

Given the unusual model of welfare regime developed in Australia, so-cial work has only played a minor and residual role in the main engine of redistribution. Nevertheless, as part of efforts to promote national recon-struction at the end of World War 2, the Commonwealth government opened up a significant role for social workers in the federally-run in-come security system (Taylor, 1947). Social work managed to firmly es-tablish itself in that context, and has retained a central role in public welfare. The nature of the Australian income security system is such that social work, by remaining centrally engaged in that system, rendered it-self important in the promotion of the Australian version of social citizen-ship rights. It is also paradoxically similarly implicated in "Workfare Oz-style."

Social work was moderately successful in positioning itself in the incrementally developed post-war arrangements for social welfare and health services in the Australian states (McDonald & Jones, 2000). In the 1950s social work developed slowly in statutory child welfare, health and disability, and to a lesser extent, corrections (Boas & Craw-ley, 1976). Nevertheless, it remained a small but distinct occupational group within a similarly small social welfare labor market. Significant expansionary opportunities presented themselves in the period of wel-fare state building in the 1970s when substantial growth in social wel-fare services occurred (Martin, 1996). In essence, the 1970s, 1980s and, to a lesser extent, the early 1990s, were the high point of Australian so-cial work within the Australian welfare state. Nevertheless, social work as an occupational group, along with welfare paraprofessionals, has continued to prosper and, interestingly, shows little sign of waning (Healy & Meagher, 2004). Furthermore, the values and aspirations of

Australian social work were, for the most part, largely congruent with those of the mature Australian welfare state.

Because of the relationship between the Commonwealth and the states, Australian social work is not as implicated in workfare-related programs as is American social work. Nevertheless, there are two primary–and in policy terms–interlinked sites where workfare is the *primary* rationality of operation. The first of these is Centrelink, the Commonwealth income security agency. The second is the Job Network–a quasi-market network of over 200 non-state organizations, for-profit and non-profit, operating in over 2,000 sites across the country providing employment services on behalf of the Federal government.

WORKFARE OZ-STYLE:
SOCIAL WORK, JOB NETWORK AND CENTRELINK

There are many perspectives that provide insights into the implications of workfare for social work: examining the profession's response as policy activists, or exploring the potential for new sites and types of social work practice that may emerge in the context of workfare. This paper focuses on the implications of workfare for the *nature* of social work. We suggest that welfare systems function as institutions in that they promote a set of norms, expectations and structures that, among other things, shape professional practices, in this instance social work (Powell & DiMaggio, 1991). Through introducing new ideas and suggesting new practices, workfare represents *institutional change* which transforms the way in which we view the nature of client problems, what social work is, what social workers do, and how they do it (Greenwood, Suddaby, & Hinings, 2002). The institutional logic of workfare provides new rules for the welfare game and shapes possible responses that are considered appropriate. Changes in an institutional logic over time lead to changes in the functioning and behavior of participants such as social workers.

Importantly, institutional change of this magnitude has been demonstrated to transform the functioning and behavior of professions considerably more powerful than social work, for example, in relation to medicine and managed care in the USA (Scott, Reuf, Mendel, & Caronna, 2000). Similarly, workfare may prove to be a profound development for social work with potential consequences for the identities and practices of social workers as they engage with it.

The Job Network

In 1996, reforms in Australian social security and employment services introduced the notion of "mutual obligation," in which the receipt of income support became subject to an obligation requirement in the form of "active job-seeking behavior." Employment policy initiatives have subsequently exhibited alignment with the "active society" orientation pursued by the OECD, characterized by a focus on the deficits of the unemployed as constitutive of the "problem" of unemployment. In 1998, the Australian Government adopted what the OECD (2001) considered to be one of the most radical experiments internationally in employment services to the unemployed–the Job Network. Replacing the long-standing government-operated labor exchange, an integrated quasi-market of employment services was created linking the purchaser (Commonwealth Department of Employment and Workplace Relations [DEWR]) with two categories of provider. One of these is Centrelink, the government income support agency, and the other is the Job Network. Job Network agencies work within formal contractual arrangements entered into with DEWR.

Job Network members provide different services to the unemployed, depending upon their assessed degree of risk and employability (McDonald, Marston, & Buckley, 2003). Those adjudged as the most employable receive basic labor exchange services provided by a networked electronic information system run by the government, accessed via remote terminals located in each Job Network outlet. Those assessed as having significant barriers to employment and/or who have been unemployed for more than 12 months are assigned to Intensive Support Customised Assistance.

Individuals fitting this category are required to work closely with a Job Network case manager. Through a range of assessments and interventions, this intensive level of assistance is designed to render an unemployed person "job ready," and to assist him or her into employment through whatever means are considered individually appropriate. Failure to engage with these prescribed activities can result in an adverse "participation report," in which a case manager reports the person to Centrelink which then imposes a regime of financial penalties in the form of deductions from income support payments.

Job Network case managers are street-level bureaucrats, embodying the logic of Workfare Oz-style. It is within the case manager-unemployed person relationship that the social relations, particularly the power relations, of Workfare Oz-style are enacted, and in which the identities of both sets of participants are shaped (Dean, 1999, 1995; Foucault, 1977). To date, there is extraordinarily limited data available at this level of observation, and even less on the experiences of social workers as case managers. Indeed, one authoritative local commentator considers Job Network agencies to be "black boxes," the inner workings of which are, at best, opaque (Considine, 2001). Nevertheless, some preliminary work does illustrate possible trends (Marston & McDonald, 2003; McDonald & Marston, 2005; Bigby & Files, 2003).

First, case managers in the Australian Job Network differentially take up and deploy the rationality or logic of workfare in their attempts to "shape" the identities of the long-term unemployed. Traditional or standard social work frameworks and approaches to practice are used, but often these are subsumed within the dominant logic of workfare. McDonald and Marston (2005) and show how case managers, using psychologically-derived frameworks or models of motivation, deploy empathetic, pedagogical and ultimately coercive authority in the case management relationship as the following examples illustrate. The first shows the use of empathetic authority to "naturalize" what is essentially a manipulative relationship:

> How we talk, how we approach somebody, our gestures and things like that, that's just a natural part of us. Our naturalness is actually one of the most important things. I think a lot of people have never had anyone to believe in them . . . I found that even the ones that have been skeptical about it, as soon as I kind of say, "I trust that you want to work and that you are doing the best that you can," it's amazing the result that happened. They hear the great things that are being said about them. Some of it may not yet be true, but it's what we hope will be true of that person, like, "They're punctual, they're enthusiastic, they're motivated." And you see them start to sit up higher in their chair and feel really good when they leave for that interview.

In many instances, empathetic authority was linked to the use of coercive authority, apparently for the purpose of legitimizing the coercive act. For example: "I find that if I have breached a client, the rapport is better and that person will get a job" (A breach refers to a negative participation report).

Bigby and Files (2003) identified the following four styles of decision-making when case managers were deciding whether or not to breach someone:

1. "Enforcers"–who demonstrated a negative view of human nature and assumed the worst of job seekers.
2. "Truth seekers"–who evinced interest in seeking the "truth" or evidence that would back up job seekers' claims.
3. "Worthiness testers"–who made judgments based on an evaluation of the morality (in terms of workfare activation) of job seeker.
4. "History seekers"–who sought information about job seekers' history and life experience, taking into account vulnerability and social disadvantage.

We suggest that the history seeker style is closest to social work. Two interesting observations can be made here. First, what appear to be social work frameworks were apparent in the range of decision-making styles (and in the frameworks of workers reported by Marston and McDonald). Second, the extent to which such frameworks follow through into active discretion on the part of case managers in their dealings with the unemployed is questionable. For example, Marston and McDonald (2003) noted that the case managers themselves were in the contractual Job Network regime and, irrespective of organizational auspice, subject to significant disciplinary measures in regards to performance outcomes.

The following extract of a case manager working in a large religious nonprofit agency involved in the Job Network (Marston & McDonald, 2005, 309) illustrates:

Case Manager 3: I don't know if you saw [the monthly performance target list] on [the office manager's] notice board?

INT: Yeah I did. . . . I noticed a distinct difference between the targets and the outcomes.

Case Manager 3: Yeah.

INT: So is this like a monthly thing?

Case Manager 3: Monthly, yep.

INT: So your targets and outcomes. What happens if you don't reach them?

Case Manager 3: Um.

INT: Sometimes you would?

Case Manager 3: Most of the time I have. I'm not out to . . . look I can't possibly reach the, the placement outcomes . . . you get all these emails [from head office], but that was exactly like [names a for-profit provider where she had been previously employed]. They're all the same [Job Network agencies]. They say they're not that driven, but that's a fine example that it is.

INT: Hmm.

Case Manager 3: Yeah, and you get, you know, the stick.

Nevertheless, it is possible that the rationalities of workfare coexist, and probably compete, with those of social work. In a preliminary analysis of the data set of 1,100 case managers, *both* rationalities were present, here expressed in case manager orientations to the unemployed:

The key to the whole unemployment problem is to MAKE PEOPLE RESPONSIBLE FOR THEIR ACTIONS. PLEASE PUT A TIME LIMIT ON THE DOLE and STOP GIVING MONEY TO YOUNG PEOPLE WHO HAVE CHILDREN FOR ALL THE WRONG REASONS.

Job Seekers know the system better than the providers!! They know their "rights." They demand; they act like spoilt children and the government lets them get away with it—when you have had someone on benefits for 15 years I think that is a sick joke! There is nothing wrong with these people; they are on a free ride and love it—they probably have a book of excuses that they all read from and use to Centrelink and their network provider. I feel that after 12 months of benefits they should be cut off—there is work but these people on benefits are supported by the government so they are choosey—if they don't like, they don't do. I feel there should be harsher rules and regulations.

And conversely:

> I am constantly trying to keep drug-affected, angry, personality-disordered or non-motivated people in the motivated head space to actually attend their jobs when I can see a poorly serviced client group being overlooked by employers. The lack of professionalism on-site is a constant problem. My colleagues do not necessarily have the skills or information to ascertain whether or not we are looking after a client with a mental illness who can't work in a team, or has medications that have side effects that present unattractively to employers.

> I understand we require the outcomes, but we are moving further and further away from helping human beings.

> I believe the present system works very well if the right staff are on board within the Network agency. I have come across [case managers] who do not genuinely care about the job seeker and this can be detrimental to both the client and the Network agency. The right staff are everything within this employment services contract. You need staff who will go the extra mile at all times.

Finally, in a comparison of Denmark and Australian employment services, similar tendencies are evident (Marston, Larson, & McDonald, 2005). The Danish case managers (who were *all* social workers) operated quite differently from many of their Australian counterparts. They were, for example, more attuned and responsive to the social and environmental issues confronting their clients, and they displayed considerably more discretion and autonomy in the way they worked. The Australian case managers, on the other hand, were significantly more constrained, and operated in a manner congruent with the institutional logic of the policy context in which they worked. They were also less able to use discretion to mitigate the effects of these policies because they themselves were subject to a range of organizational performance measures that focused on achieving certain output targets. Further, with some notable exceptions, their modes of working tended to unambiguously locate the cause of unemployment firmly within the personality and psyche of the unemployed person.

These important differences in part reflect the political and cultural orientations of a social democratic Denmark and a largely residual Neo-liberal Australian welfare state. However, at this stage it is presumptuous to suggest that these differences simply represent practices conforming to dominant principles and rationalities of each country. At the level of policy discourse, while there is a degree of convergence taking place between these two very different welfare models, Marston, Larson, and McDonald (2005) suggest that this is not automatically reflected in the practice of case management and that the reality is far more nuanced. Nevertheless, these initial findings suggest that, in the context of contemporary workfare, a focus on abstract typologies or ideal types is not all that helpful in getting the measure of workfare. In the case of workfare and social work there is probably more ambiguity, incoherence and contradiction than is suggested by linear accounts of workfare policies and programs, which often assume that welfare provision and social work practice are becoming progressively more (il)-liberal. The ambiguities inherent in social work practice under conditions of workfare are revealed in the case of Centrelink.

Centrelink

Centrelink is the key government agency overseeing Workfare Oz-style and is the primary gateway into the Job Network. It is, at a minimum, an interesting agency. Established in 1941 as the Department of Social Services, it was later renamed as the Department of Social Security (DSS), and finally, in 1997, it was transformed into Centrelink. This latter transformation was radical in terms of Australian public administration (Rowlands, 1999), as well as important for our purposes here. Centrelink is the preeminent example of New Public Management-inspired reform in Australia. Institutionalizing a form of purchaser-provider split, Centrelink is the primary service delivery agency of the Commonwealth Government, providing services on a contractual basis on behalf of an array of government "client" departments and agencies. Centrelink, because of its role in determining eligibility for various forms of social assistance (and the conditions that attach to them), is, nevertheless, a one-stop-shop monopoly (Keating, 2001). While Centrelink provides services *to* Australians, it is vital to remember that its clients are *government entities*, a design feature which in one stroke dissolves any vestige of income security as social rights of citizenship which might have adhered to DSS clients under the old regime.

In governance terms, Centrelink was, until recently, an independent statutory authority operating under a government-appointed board. The board consisted of seven members–a chairman, three members drawn from private industry, two Directors General from the main client departments (who had no voting rights), and the Chief Executive Officer (Mulgan, 2003). The original structure (and the significance of the private sector board members) was to promote cultural change, particularly at the interface between the organization and the various categories of claimants. More recently, Centrelink has been reabsorbed into the federal bureaucracy and is now part of a new Department of Human Services. The driving rationale under both models is a desire by government to improve the *effectiveness* as well as the efficiency of service delivery. Adopting the language and style of the private sector, Centrelink management incorporated the latest devices for improving performance, for example, benchmarking and the "balanced scorecard." Welfare beneficiaries have become "customers" served by "customer service officers" (formerly "counter staff"). Offices were redesigned and an extensive array of "customer satisfaction" procedures were introduced, such as the "value creation workshops" (ANAO, 2005), citizens' charters, and so forth. The real efficiencies made by Centrelink have been through the extensive deployment of information and communications technologies. Given the size and complexity[1] of the enterprise, there was little choice.[2]

Centrelink has employed social workers for the last 60 years. There are at least 600 social workers in social work-designated positions and a significant number in non-designated management positions (Fitzgibbon & Hargraves, 2001). In earlier versions of the agency the social work role was documented, for example, in a paper to the very first Australian Conference on Social Work. Lyra Taylor, the first social worker appointed, said that social workers were employed to provide a "skilled casework service to the department's beneficiaries, to make the department's administration as humane as possible, and to form a useful instrument for social progress by assembling evidence on social questions" (Fitzgibbon & Hargraves, 2001, p. 123).

Further, a community liaison and community service development role was articulated and extended in the 1960s and 1970s. Following a series of reviews, designated social workers were more closely articulated with the core business of the agency–income maintenance–but not in the sense of involvement in claimant eligibility determination. In 1996, the social work role was described as:

> To promote the wellbeing of Departmental clients by working towards the social justice objective of preventing and relieving hardship and suffering . . . to promote and facilitate the access of clients to Departmental income support programs and community

resources . . . to provide supportive social work services to Departmental clients in situations of crisis and distress; to promote and facilitate the sensitive delivery of the Department's services to clients; and promote and facilitate the development of income support and community services to meet the needs of Departmental clients. (Department of Social Security, 1996: 1)

In essence, the pre-Centrelink social work role had five dimensions:

1. Facilitating client access to benefits through internal advocacy,
2. Providing brief casework and referral services,
3. Facilitating the development of supportive services in local communities *outside* of Centrelink,
4. Improving overall service delivery through developmental work with Departmental staff and processes,
5. Providing input to Departmental (and Government) policy development.

Of interest is what has changed. The transformation into Centrelink created new demands for all participants, and social workers were no exceptions. In 1998, the social workers were obliged to submit a "service offer" to the Centrelink "guiding coalition" about what they could contribute to the new organization. In this offer, the Centrelink social workers did two things. Utilizing the language of the new organization, they first re-badged a large part of their traditional role and second, identified at least two major "spaces" for practice and quickly established competence in those fields.

In regard to the first response, the social workers have been able to capitalize on, or succumb to, the "new language," representing the new institutional rationality of Centrelink. As Rose (1999) suggests, the discourses of Centrelink contain some very predictable discursive artifacts such as: life events and life transitions, personalized solutions, effective networks, enterprise practices, empowerment and community partnerships.

In articulating the design for the new Centrelink, such terms or artifacts were promoted by the "guiding coalition" as key features of the new institutional rationality of Centrelink. For social work these same phrases have the capacity to pick up traditional professional notions and frameworks. As a consequence, the social workers were able to couch their "offer" within the discursive framework of the new institutional rationality. The "new" roles articulated by the social workers are:

1. To provide casework services in the early phase of life transition to Centrelink customers who are most at risk of harm or abuse, exclusion from the labor market, poverty or social isolation;
2. To work with customers, their families and other human service organizations to develop personalized solutions and service plans with the aim to promote independence;
3. To work with community agencies to develop and sustain the most efficient and effective network of human services for Centrelink customers;
4. *To work with community agencies, recognized experts and Centrelink staff to develop high quality service in community recovery situations following disasters;*
5. To share values, knowledge and skills with staff in customer service outlets to assist them to engage with customers to provide personalized and effective labor market and income support options and solutions, and;
6. To work to develop and implement training and development strategies to achieve effective cultural change and excellence in customer service (Fitzgibbon, 2000, p. 183).

The fourth role represents an existing role more highly prioritized in recent times. Thus, older roles were subsumed within the new, and wherever possible, the social workers demonstrated *excellence* in what they did, for example, brief casework in relation to young homeless people (Squires & Kramaric-Trojak, 2003).

The second major response was the development of new "spaces" of practice. The most influential of these is social work practice in the call centers (Humphries & Camilleri, 2002) where, despite the efficiency benchmarks dictating time-limited calls for the bulk of operatives, social workers have been able to demonstrate the value of longer, more in-depth calls.

So what do these developments represent in terms of the future of social work in Workfare Oz-style? Does it represent discursive transformation through the insidious and pervasive effect of immersion in the new discourse or institutional rationality of Centrelink? Or, as Healey et al. (2003, 67) suggest, will engagement with alternative discourses not necessarily lead to the eventual defeat of a specific social work rationality? Phillips, Lawrence, and Hardy (2004) suggest that the linkages between discourses (rationalities) and the formation of new or alternative institutions are far more nuanced than previously theoretically imagined. Ultimately this is an empirical question to which there are no substantive answers as yet but some interesting possibilities.

CONCLUSION

We suggest that Workfare Oz-style has significant implications for Australian social work, and that the local quarantine effect to the Job Network and Centrelink is not likely to last. Given recent political events, Workfare Oz-style is set to play out across the welfare sector more broadly and Australian social workers currently operating in seemingly unaffected contexts will be drawn into the institutional logic of workfare. We also conclude that, because of the pervasiveness of New Public Management-inspired refashioning of social welfare service delivery, when Workfare Oz-style does spread it will not appear as alien or objectionable as many would like to believe.

Our deliberations to date actually pose more questions than answers. Specifically, does workfare represent institutional change? If so, will social work survive? And, if so, in what form? We tentatively conclude that it will, but we are less clear about its future form or, more precisely, its future rationality. Further, if we accept that there is such a thing as an international professional project of social work, such questions apply to all contexts where workfare is being enacted and not just to Australia. Finally, we suggest that the impact of workfare on the *ontological status* of social work remains a field wide-open for empirical investigation.

NOTES

1. On a typical day, Centrelink IT supports 55,000 business function points in 14 million lines of code through 8,000 functions on 3,200 screens to 31,000 desktops and 400 LAN servers, in 1000 sites. This means that 13,000 users concurrently generate 12 million online transactions each day on 14 million customer records (Vardon, 2003).

2. For example, Centrelink has 1000 sites of service delivery, including 28 call centres, 25,000 staff, 6.4 million "customers," 70 different products and services, 232 million payments a year (around A$50 billion), with 100 million letters sent to customers, 6.5 million home visits, 20 million office appointments and 30 million web site hits (Vardon, 2001).

REFERENCES

Australian National Audit Office (ANAO) (2005). *Centrelink's Value Creation Program.* Canberra: Australian National Audit Office.

Bigby, C., & Files, W. (2003). Street-level leniency or unjust inconsistency? An examination of breach recommendation decision making in a for-profit job network agency. *Australian Journal of Labour Economics, 6*(2), 277-291.

Boas, P.J., & Crawley, J. (1976). *Social Work in Australia*. Sydney: Australia International Press.

Cass, B. (1986). *The Case for Review of the Australian Social Security System*. Canberra: Department of Social Security.

Castles, F.G. (1983). *The Working Class and Welfare*. Sydney: Allen and Unwin.

Considine, M. (2001). *Enterprising States: The Public Management of Welfare to Work*. Melbourne: Cambridge University Press.

Dean, M. (1999). *Governmentality: Power and Rule in Modern Society*. London: Sage.

Dean, M. (1995). Governing the unemployed self in active society. *Economy and Society, 24*(4), 559-583.

Department of Social Security (1996). *Social Work Handbook*. Canberra: Australian Government Publishing Service.

Finn, D. (1999). Job guarantees for the unemployed: Lessons from Australian welfare reform. *Journal of Social Policy, 28*(1), 53-71.

Fitzgibbon, P. (2000). Social work and the human services in a corporatised environment: The case of Centrelink. In I. O'Connor, P. Smyth, & J. Warburton (Eds.), *Contemporary Perspectives on Social Work and the Human Services: Challenges and Change*. Sydney: Longman, pp. 176-189.

Fitzgibbon, D., & Hargraves, D. (2001). Social work in the field of income maintenance. In M. Alston & J. McKinnon (Eds.), *Social Work: Fields of Practice*. Sydney: Oxford University Press, pp. 122-135.

Foucault, M. (1977). *Discipline and Punish: The Birth of the Prison*. London: Allen Lane.

Gilbert, N. (2002). *Transformation of the Welfare State: The Silent Surrender of Public Responsibility*. New York: Oxford University Press.

Glennerster, H. (1999). Which welfare states are most likely to survive? *International Social Welfare, 8*(1), 2-13.

Greenwood, R., Suddaby, R., & Hinings, C.R. (2002). Theorising change: The role of professional asssociations in the transformation of institutional fields. *Academy of Management Journal, 43*(1), 58-79.

Healey, P., de Magalhaes, C., Madanipour, A., & Pendlebury, J. (2003). Place, identity and local politics: Analysing initiatives in deliberative governance. In M. Hajer & H. Wagenaar (Eds.), *Deliberative Policy Analysis: Understanding Governance in the Network Society*. Cambridge: Cambridge University Press, pp. 60-87.

Healy, K., & Meagher, G. (2004). The reprofessionalisation of social work: Collaborative approaches for achieving professional recognition. *British Journal of Social Work, 34*(2), 243-260.

Humphries, P., & Camilleri, P. (2002). Social work and technology: Challenges for social workers in practice: A case study. *Australian Social Work, 55*(4), 251-259.

Jessop, B. (2002). *The Future of the Capitalist State*. Cambridge: Polity Press.

Keating, M. (2001). Reshaping service delivery. In G. Davis & P. Weller (Eds.), *Are You Being Served: States, Citizens and Governance*. Sydney: Allen and Unwin, pp. 98-125.

Keating, P. (1994). *Working Nation: Policies and Programs*. Canberra: Australian Government Publishing Service.

Marston, G., & McDonald, C. (2003). The psychology, ethics and social relations of unemployment. *Australian Journal of Labour Economics, 6*(2), 293-315.

Marston, G., Larson, J.E., & McDonald, C. (2005). *The Active Subjects of Welfare Reform: A Comparative Study of Employment Services in Australia and Denmark*. Unpublished manuscript.

Martin, E. (1996). An update on census data: Good news for social work? *Australian Social Work, 49*(2), 29-36.

McDonald, C., & Marston, G. (2005). Workfare as welfare: Governing unemployment in the advanced liberal state. *Critical Social Policy, 25*(3), 374-401.

McDonald, C., Marston, G., & Buckley, A. (2003). Risk technology in Australia: The role of the job seeker classification instrument. *Critical Social Policy, 23*(4), 498-525.

McDonald, C., & Jones, A. (2000). Reconstructing and reconceptualising social work in the emerging milieu. *Australian Social Work, 53*(3), 3-11.

Mulgan, R. (2003). Centrelink: A new approach to service delivery. In C. Aspalter (Ed.), *Neoliberalism and the Australian Welfare State*. Hong Kong: Casa Verde Publishing, pp. 169-180.

Organization for Economic Cooperation and Development (2001). *Innovations in Labour Market Policies: The Australian Way*. Paris: OECD.

Osborne, D., & Gaebler, T. (1992). *Reinventing Government*. Reading, MA: Addison-Wesley.

Peters, G. (1996). *The Future of Governing: Four Emerging Models*. Lawrence, KS: University Press of Kansas.

Phillips, N., Lawrence, T.B., & Hardy, C. (2004). Discourse and institutions. *Academy of Management Review, 29*(4), 635-652.

Powell, W.W., & DiMaggio, P.J. (Eds.) (1991). *The New Institutionalism in Organizational Analysis*. Chicago: University of Chicago Press.

Rose, N. (1999). *Powers of Freedom: Reframing Political Thought*. Cambridge: Cambridge University Press.

Rowlands, D. (1999). Institutional change in the Australian public service–The case of DSS and Centrelink. *Australian Social Policy, 1*: 183-201.

Scott, W.R., Reuf, M., Mendel, P., & Caronna, C. (2000). *Institutional Change and Healthcare Organizations: From Professional Dominance to Managed Care*. Chicago: University of Chicago Press.

Smyth, P., & Cass, B. (1998). *Contesting the Australian Way: States, Markets and Civil Society*. Cambridge: Cambridge University Press.

Squires, J., & Kramaric-Trojak, N. (2003). Centrelink: How social workers make a difference for young persons. A model of intervention. *Australian Social Work, 56*(4), 293-304.

Taylor, L. (1947). Social work in statutory agencies. In *Proceedings of the First Australian Conference of Social Work*. Sydney: Australian Association of Social Workers.

Turner, G. (1995). Whatever happened to national identity? Film and the nation in the 1990s. *Metro, 100*(summer), 32-35.

Vardon, S. (2003). Managing change: The Centrelink experience. *Canberra Bulletin of Public Administration, 107*, 35-40.

Vardon, S. (2001). *Trust Us–We're from Centrelink*. Paper given to the Queensland Division of the Institute of Public Administration, Australia Annual State Conference, August 24.

Wearing, M. (1994). Disclaiming citizenship? Social rights, social justice and welfare in the 1990s. In M. Wearing & R. Berreen (Eds.), *Welfare and Social Policy in Australia: The Distribution of Advantage*. Sydney: Harcourt Brace, pp. 177-198.

Recent Developments in Welfare to Work in Hong Kong: Opportunities for Social Work

Kwong-leung Tang

SUMMARY. The Asian financial crisis (1997) has created a social care crisis resulting in rising unemployment, poverty, income inequalities and homelessness. Although faced with dwindling public finances, the Hong Kong Special Administrative Region (SAR) government had been compelled to tackle these problems. However, it has been attracted to the neo-liberal recipe: changing the subvention system to a block grant, curbing social spending, and tightening eligibility for social assistance. Notably, the introduction of the Intensive Employment Assistance Projects (IEAPs), which are the first welfare to work programs in East Asia, has become a major policy tool. This paper reports on a study of the impact of the projects, one of the key pillars for welfare to work programs. The IEAPs were found to have brought about positive changes in welfare clients' motivation to work and sense of self-reliance. Social workers from both traditional and progressive NGOs have etched, in various

Kwong-leung Tang, PhD, is Professor of Social Work, Chinese University of Hong Kong, T.C. Cheng Building, United College, The Chinese University of Hong Kong, Shatin, New Territories, Hong Kong (E-mail: kltang@cuhk.edu.hk).

[Haworth co-indexing entry note]: "Recent Developments in Welfare to Work in Hong Kong: Opportunities for Social Work." Tang, Kwong-leung. Co-published simultaneously in *Journal of Policy Practice* (The Haworth Press, Inc.) Vol. 5. No. 2/3, 2006, pp. 129-147; and: *International Perspectives on Welfare to Work Policy* (ed: Richard Hoefer, and James Midgley) The Haworth Press, Inc., 2006, pp. 129-147. Single or multiple copies of this article are available for a fee from The Haworth Document Delivery Service [1-800- HAWORTH, 9:00 a.m. - 5:00 p.m. (EST). E-mail address: docdelivery@ haworthpress.com].

ways, their place in the welfare to work programs and contributed to the debate on welfare reform in Hong Kong. *[Article copies available for a fee from The Haworth Document Delivery Service: 1-800-HAWORTH. E-mail address: <docdelivery@haworthpress.com> Website: <http://www.HaworthPress. com> © 2006 by The Haworth Press, Inc. All rights reserved.]*

KEYWORDS. Welfare to work, welfare reform, Hong Kong, Intensive Employment Assistance Projects

THE EAST ASIAN ECONOMIC CRISIS

The Asian financial crisis of 1997 shattered the prosperity of many wealthy East Asian countries. Prior to the crisis, economic growth of the tiger economies of Hong Kong, Taiwan, South Korea and Singapore had been particularly spectacular: GDP per capita rose in Hong Kong from around US$2,400 in 1965 to US$12,000 in the early 1990s while GDP per capita income in South Korea increased from about US$600 to more than US$5,000. This rapid rate of growth continued during the first half of the 1990s when average annual rates of GDP growth consistently exceeded 5% per annum, exceeding the growth records of the world's industrial nations such as Britain, Canada, Sweden and the United States (Tang, 2000a). For the tiger economies, low unemployment, rapid economic development and high inflation were the order of the day.

Decades of rapid economic development made Asian nations complacent; they believed that economic development alone would ultimately eliminate all forms of social problems. As a result, they did not formulate coherent social policies and relied on strong cultural and familial obligations to meet social needs (Tang & Midgley, 2002). Despite the use of free market rhetoric to characterize their approach, East Asian governments actively engaged in promoting social protection to meet rising expectations on the part of the public and to gain public support (Chow, 2003; Tang & Midgley, 2002; Goodman et al., 1998).

The case of Hong Kong is illustrative of this trend. Colonial rule had been characterized by a residual approach in social care until the onset of the 1966-67 riots. Immediately after the riots, Governor MacLehose introduced a comprehensive plan for social reform, giving center stage to housing, education, medical and health, and social welfare. In the area of social welfare, public assistance and social allowances for the disabled and the elderly were introduced. A number of other policy documents were produced (White Papers on Youth, the Elderly, and Rehabilitation). A new social welfare planning machinery was introduced: the Five Year Plan setting out the policy objectives governing the provision and future development of social welfare services and the specific targets of expansion for each service area. New social welfare services programs were later put in place in 1977: school social work, outreach youth services, special services for the disabled and the elderly (Tang, 1998).

Since then, the Hong Kong colonial government had adopted an incremental approach to social welfare in which social programs evolved in an *ad hoc* fashion, haphazardly emulated Western developments, or perpetuated programs introduced during colonial times (Tang & Midgley, 2002; Midgley, 1986). When the colonial government implemented these welfare measures, there was considerable policy transfer and diffusion of ideas from advanced industrialized countries. Toward the end of the 1990s, East Asian countries were presented with a new and tough social and economic situation. The precipitating factor was the Asian financial crisis of 1997 that brought a serious impact on most of the economies of the East Asian region. Most of them were haunted by the problems of unemployment, poverty, income inequalities and homelessness.

Hong Kong was ill prepared for the Asian financial crisis since there was a lack of adequate social protection. As noted, Hong Kong colonial government neither formulated coherent social policies nor created comprehensive social welfare programs. This policy legacy was not abandoned when Tung Chee-hwa (the Chief Executive) took up the leadership of the post-colonial government. Social welfare expansion in colonial Hong Kong had, in the main, been built upon rapid economic growth. After the 1997 crisis, the economic pain was felt by most people. Some socioeconomic indicators bear this out. The unemployment rate in Hong Kong reached 6.7% in March 2002 and hit the record high 8.6% during the SARS crisis in early 2003. In terms of income distribution, the Gini coefficient for the city-state reached a record of 0.525 in 2001. Many more people have applied for public assistance and income disparities have worsened. Worse still, Hong Kong had been bombarded with crisis after crisis, starting with the Asian financial crisis. More recently, the SARS (severe acute respiratory syndrome) crisis led to a rapidly declining economy.

Attracted to the neo-liberal idea of "small government, big market" and its consequent managerialism, the Hong Kong Special Administrative Region (SAR) government responded to the crisis in the following ways: changing the subvention system to a block grant, curbing social spending, and tightening eligibility for social assistance. Above all, welfare to work programs were introduced in 1999, which can be considered as the first of their kind in East Asia. This paper looks at the Intensive Employment Assistance Projects (IEAPs) (2003-07), one of the most current welfare-to-work programs, and assesses its impacts on welfare clients as well as the role of professional social workers. We argue that social workers have an important role to play in the process of poverty alleviation.

RESPONDING TO THE CRISIS

Facing economic and social challenges after 1997, the Hong Kong SAR government held on to its long-standing belief that increasing social spending in bad economic times would only undermine the prospect of economic recovery. After the 1997 crisis, the government took the view that economic recovery was not far away and painted a rosy picture of the future. Measures were taken to assist businesses and the middle class to weather the storm. But the crisis deepened, and the challenge looked daunting to the SAR government. Economically, its fiscal deficits ballooned. More people were laid off. As Hong Kong did not have any unemployment insurance, the unemployed had to apply for social assistance (called "Comprehensive Social Security Assistance" [CSSA]). This rapidly boosted the number of people on welfare from about 88,600 cases in the mid-1990s to 235,700 cases in 1999. This unprecedented increase in spending on social assistance alarmed the government and there was a growing fear that a "culture of dependency" would emerge among those receiving benefits (Tang, 2000b; Social Welfare Department, 2005).

In response to the growing numbers receiving benefits, the SAR government sought to limit social assistance eligibility in 1998-99. First, it reduced the benefit rate for larger families. Standard social assistance rates for able-bodied adults were reduced by 10% for three-person households and 20% for those households with more than three persons. Additionally, the government tightened eligibility criteria so that fewer people would apply. As social welfare spending continued to soar, these measures were followed by another round of reduction in CSSA payments in 2004. At the same time, a new population policy (2004) excluded newly arrived people from the welfare system. The new policy required CSSA applicants to be Hong Kong residents for at least seven years before they were eligible to apply for financial assistance.

Hong Kong's responses to the crisis marked the influence of neo-liberal thinking which appealed to the territory's political leaders. With the onset of the welfare state crisis in the mid-1970s, the neo-liberal paradigm has become increasingly dominant in many advanced industrialized countries (Midgley, 1997). Neo-liberal social and labor-market policy combines objectives of the dismantling of welfare and the roll-back of entitlements with an insistent focus on the activation and enforcement of work (Peck, 2002). These ideas were championed by international organizations (the International Monetary Fund [IMF], the World Bank, and the Asian Development Bank) that supported the adoption of neo-liberal economic policies (IMF, 1999). The IMF argued that the best strategy for recovery required the adoption of macroeconomic policies that reduced government intervention and deregulated the economy. In the area of social care, it strongly emphasized "cost-effective" social programs that would not create market disincentives.

It has to be noted that there are other international organizations that offered alternative policy prescriptions to the crisis-struck Asian nations. Among them, the ILO's (1999) recommendation stood out. It took an active role in promoting the social protection approach to social policy in the region by sending its delegation to crisis-struck Asian nations. It recommended that they adopt comprehensive social protection programs, employment creation and proactive labor market policies, and ratify or better implement the ILO's various conventions that deal with social security and related programs (Tang & Midgley, 2002; Cooney, 1999; Holtz, 1999; ILO, 1999; Fraser & Nyland, 1997).

SUPPORT FOR SELF-RELIANCE PROGRAM (SFS)

Hong Kong as discussed earlier was facing a paradox immediately after the Asian crisis: fiscal challenge together with a swelling pressure on welfare rolls. In the eyes of the post-colonial government, it was necessary to find some means to tackle the rising caseload of social assistance. Total welfare spending in Hong Kong has been on the rise. In 2003-04, the estimated expenditure for social welfare programs was HK$32,869 million (US$1 = HK$7.8). This represented an increase of 4.9% over the actual expenditure of HK$31,348 million of 2002-03. At the same time, Hong Kong witnessed exorbitant increases in CSSA cases after the Asian financial crisis, rising from 186,932 cases in 1997 to 295,694 at the end of 2004 (Table 1) (Commission on Poverty, 2005). The average growth in the number of cases per annum is 10.9%. Yet, about one third of the CSSA cases are able-bodied welfare recipients (single parents, low earnings and unemployment) who are capable of work (Table 2 for single parents). The annual growth rates of able-bodied cases (single parents, low earnings and unemployment) are 20.7%, 32.8% and 25.0% respectively. To the government, the only way to reduce CSSA spending appeared to be the promotion of these capable recipients' work involvement and thereby self-reliance. This concern was a basis for the shift from a social provision approach to a welfare to work

TABLE 1. The CSSA Scheme: Number of CSSA Cases by Nature of Case (1997-2004)

Year	Old age	Permanent disability	Temporary disability/ill health	Single parent	Low earnings	Unemployment	Others	Total
1997	109,150	12,801	20,438	15,849	4,148	16,976	7,570	186,932
1998	121,778	14,932	25,089	24,595	7,348	30,290	3,422	227,454
1999	133,613	11,732	19,964	25,467	8,008	28,085	3,821	230,681
2000	134,230	12,243	19,800	25,902	8,432	23,573	3,880	228,060
2001	138,232	13,522	19,705	28,504	9,008	28,886	3,816	241,673
2002	142,762	14,717	20,847	33,156	10,607	40,513	3,941	266,571
2003	147,032	15,697	22,198	37,301	13,534	50,118	4,326	290,206
2004	148,821	16,764	23,201	39,536	16,176	43,231	4,965	295,694
Average growth per annum (1997-2004)	7.9%	7.7%	7.9%	20.7%	32.8%	25.0%	1.8%	10.9

Note: Figures refer to those as at the end of the year.
Source: Adapted from Commission on Poverty (2005), Annex A.

TABLE 2. The CSSA Scheme: Year-End Figures of All Cases and Single Parent Cases for the Years 1997-98 to 2003-04

Financial year	Year-end number of single parent cases	Year-on-year change of single parent cases (%)	% share of all CSSA cases	Year-end number of all CSSA cases	Year-on-year change of all CSSA cases (%)
1997-98	17,161	+29.0	8.8	195,645	+17.3
1998-99	25,613	+49.3	11.0	232,819	+19.0
1999-2000	25,146	−1.8	11.0	228,015	−2.1
2000-01	26,078	+3.7	11.4	228,263	+0.1
2001-02	29,534	+13.3	11.9	247,192	+8.3
2002-03	34,249	+16.0	12.6	271,893	+10.0
2003-04	37,949	+10.8	13.1	290,705	+6.9
Average year-on-year change (1993-94 to 2003-04)	−	+20.0	−	−	+11.8

Source: Adapted from the Legislative Council Panel on Welfare Services (Subcommittee on review of the CSSA) (2005b), Annex 1.

approach. This approach continued to intensify measures to support self-reliance to help able-bodied welfare recipients to engage in work.

Other than the welfare reduction measures mentioned earlier, a review of the Comprehensive Social Security Assistance Scheme (CSSA) by the Social Welfare Department (SWD) in 1997 concluded that the implementation of the "Support for Self-reliance Scheme" (SFS) was necessary (Social Welfare Department, 2001). Under this new framework for social assistance, recipients of assistance had obligations to move from welfare to work, if they were able-bodied. Social assistance in Hong Kong was thus cast as a temporary support, a means of last-resort for those unable to support themselves, and placed a stronger emphasis on individual responsibility and the necessity and importance of work for those who were able to do so (Social Welfare Department, 2005).

Program-wise, SFS had three components: active employment assistance, community work programs, and disregarded earnings. Firstly, the active employment assistance (AEA) was introduced: the provision of personalized service to encourage and help the unemployed recipients to find work. Secondly, able-bodied people on welfare were required to participate in "volunteer projects" (i.e., Community Work Programme). Thirdly, there was the provision of disregarded earnings to serve as a reward for people moving from welfare to work (Table 3).

Across nations, an important theme of welfare to work programs is the promotion of self-reliance and self-empowerment in public assistance recipients and low-income people (Morgen & Maskovsky, 2003). Accordingly, welfare to work and self-reliance are intended to establish

TABLE 3. Support for Self-Reliance Scheme, Hong Kong (1998-2005)

Year	Programme
1998	(1) Active Employment Assistance Programme (2) Community Work Programme (3) Disregarded Earnings
2001	Intensive Employment Assistance Fund
2001	Special Job Attachment Programme
2002	Ending Exclusion Programme
2003	Intensive Employment Assistance Projects (IEAPs having 105 projects): Batch 1 (40 projects) October 2003 thru September 2004
2004	Batch 2 (30 projects) October 2004 thru September 2005
2005	Batch 3 (45 projects) October 2005 thru September 2007

a healthy life in the needy in order to upgrade their participation in the society. Furthermore, workfare and self-reliance serve to erode welfare dependency and sustain an active labor market and a reintegrated society (Noel, 1995). On the other hand, welfare to work programs share the belief that welfare recipients are capable of self-reliance and self-disciplining (Peck, 2001). The programs also contribute to the integration of society and the eradication of social exclusion (Dahl, 2003).

It is clear that the SAR government intended to instill the idea of welfare to work as a condition of receiving their welfare entitlements. Consequently, the SFS was implemented to encourage and assist unemployed CSSA recipients to regain employment and move towards self-reliance.

To step up this work ethic ideology, the SWD secured $43 million from the Legislative Council to implement a Promoting Self-Reliance Strategy in 2001. It was comprised of two projects: the Special Job Attachment (SJA) Programme and the Intensive Employment Assistance (IEA) Fund. However, these two programs were not satisfactory. Until May 2003, 42.1% of the SJA and 40.7% of the IEA participants successfully found a job, of which 49.4% and 55.3% respectively could secure only part-time employment. As for the CSSA status, 42.1% of the SJA and 68% of the IEA participants still remained trapped in the unemployment category of the CSSA net, while 30.9% and 14.4% respectively experienced a change of status from unemployment to low earnings category within the CSSA net, with a remainder of 27% and 17.6% of the participants gaining successful exit from the CSSA net. Furthermore, it was concluded that the scheme has a low cost-benefit: the operational cost is higher than the expenditure saved from the CSSA payment for the participants who could successfully exit the social security safety net (SWD, 2005).

To further promote and enhance the self-reliance ideology, the SWD launched the Ending Exclusion Project (EEP) starting March 2002, targeted at helping and encouraging CSSA single parents, whose youngest child was below age 15, to increase their social and economic participation in society to reduce the risk of social exclusion. An evaluation was conducted and its results were released in December 2003 (Leung, Ip, & Au, 2003). In this study, a longitudinal survey methodology with a control group design was employed. In comparison with the control group, EEP participants engaged in more part-time employment, exhibited more job-seeking behavior, experienced less social isolation, were able to cope more rationally, and their children had a more positive perception of the parent-child relationship. Despite these positive program effects, the EEP group obtained far less support from significant others in job-seeking than the control group.

LAUNCHING OF THE IEAPS

In 2003, the SWD implemented the latest and perhaps the most important welfare to work program. It secured funding of US$25.6 million from the Lotteries Fund and the Hong Kong Jockey Club Charities Trust to commission non-governmental organizations (NGOs) to launch 105 IEAPs by three batches in four years from October 2003 to September 2007. To distinguish it from Active Employment Assistance (AEA), also maintained by the SWD, the IEAP offers more services, including training, counseling, job matching, and post-employment support. As one of the intensified measures to strengthen the promotion of "welfare to work" and "self-reliance," the main objective of these projects is to encourage and assist members of the vulnerable groups, especially employable CSSA recipients, to return to the work force or move up the job ladder to achieve self-sufficiency, through activities such as job matching, job skills training, employment counseling, post-employment support and short-term "temporary financial aid" (designed to help recipients to tide over short-term financial hardship or to meet employment-related expenses).

Program Characteristics. The IEAPs displayed a number of characteristics: First, they aimed at not only helping the able-bodied unemployed CSSA recipients back to work but have also extended the target recipients to the near CSSA recipients so as to prevent them from falling into the CSSA net. The CSSA recipients are mandatory participants, who have been enrolled in the AEA program within three months and then referred to join these IEAPs by the SWD, whereas the near CSSA recipients are mostly voluntary participants.

Second, the government stipulated that outcome-based performance indicators are drawn up to monitor the performance of each IEAP. The minimum performance standards for each project per implementation year are as follows: (i) rendering service to no fewer than 100 participants, of whom at least 70% must be CSSA participants; (ii) assisting at least 63 CSSA participants to complete the range of activities organized; (iii) assisting at least 28 CSSA and 12 Near-CSSA participants to take up full-time employment; and (iv) assisting at least 21 CSSA participants to sustain full-time paid employment for at least three months with their status changed to either "off CSSA" or "CSSA low-earners."

Third, the IEAPs represent an intensive form of welfare to work program designed to discourage reliance on social assistance, as was done in a number of advanced industrialized countries. It can be distinguished from the active employment assistance program maintained by the SWD in that the IEAPs offer more intensive and personal services, including training, counseling, non-job-related counseling, job matching, and post-employment support, to participants.

Fourth, there is much flexibility for the NGOs in program design. To be eligible to submit an application, a NGO should be a bona fide non-profit-making agency with at least two years' experience in providing employment assistance to client groups in Hong Kong. The NGOs had the discretion to design their own projects, which could range from individualized employment counseling to setting up small-scale businesses. In addition, the NGOs are entitled to administer the temporary financial aid, which amounts to HK$200,000 annually, to provide timely financial assistance to meet the needs of the unemployed/low-income families who are not on CSSA.

Case Illustration. The International Social Service Hong Kong Branch, an agency that historically deals with overseas adoption, successfully bid for one IEAP in 2003 (ISSHKB, 2005). Within one year, some 186 CSSA recipients were recruited, over 90% of users being referred by the Hong Kong SAR government. Its IEAP was tailor-made and designed according to each trait and need of every participant. According to their own estimate, there were 66 participants who successfully secured full-time, part-time and temporary employment within the six months of the IEAPs. Major sources of work placement included food and service industries (cleaning, personal care, office work, restaurant work and technical support). To their staff, two program components were considered important in affecting the outcome: (1) actively building up a network with local employers of small-scale and cooperative business; and (2) the use of temporary financial aid which was offered to IEAP participants to tide them over temporary hardship and meet their short-term basic needs.

IMPACTS OF THE IEAPS

The IEAPs are the latest in a series of first-ever welfare to work programs in Asia after the financial crisis. The projects basically use a work-first plus approach: getting the recipients into employment through a number of measures as quickly as possible. They use a tripartite partnership model whereby private sector, government and NGOs are involved. A variety of NGOs were involved, including both traditional and progressive social service agencies. Interestingly, the Society for Community Organization, one of the leading progressive NGOs, has been praised by the SAR government in their efforts to implement successfully their IEAPs.

A distinguishing feature of these projects is the critical inputs of professional social workers. Social workers in Hong Kong have been engaged in various practice settings. However, the IEAPs now allow many of them to venture into some relatively new areas of practice and assume new roles: poverty and employment assistance. The IEAPs are not designed according to a "one-size-fits-all" model. As there is no one fixed program format for the IEAPs, social workers now serve as the IEAP program initiator and case manager, serving welfare clients in their own local community. Staff commitment is pronounced in the IEAPs, in which social workers could serve as role models for participants to learn about self-reliance and working. In giving support to their clients, social workers also have to act as a broker between different partners: business, government and NGOs. It is not unusual to see IEAP workers contacting employers and accompanying their clients for job interviews. Some of them do give post-employment support to their clients.

Finally, social workers have to continuously monitor their own projects, playing the role of a program evaluator. In assessing the impacts of their own programs on poverty reduction and welfare to work, they become a willing contributor to the welfare reform debate in Hong Kong. This was evident when all the NGOs running the IEAPs were invited to the Legislative Council in June 2005 to give their own views of the program. Some 20 NGOs did send their delegates to this meeting and invariably, all were positive of the implementation of the IEAPs. A few of them had worries at the start (e.g., worries whether their intervention in employment assistance would be effective). Outside the legislature, social workers are engaged in some form of community advocacy when airing their views of how welfare to work programs could be bettered in light of their experiences in running the IEAPs. What has been the impact of the IEAPs? According to official statistics, one may note some positive results. In the first batch of 40 projects (running from October 2003 to September 2004), 35 of the 40 projects met the performance standards set out by the government. Statistically, for this batch of 40 projects, a total of 6,245 participants were recruited. Among them, 4,778 (76.5%) were CSSA recipients and 1,467 (23.5%) were near-CSSA recipients. As of May 2005, a total of 70 IEAPs (batch 1 and 2 together) were undertaken, enrolling a total of 12,236 CSSA participants and 3,213 near-CSSA participants. Some 3,990 (32.6%) of the CSSA participants who have joined the projects could either get out of the CSSA net or reduce their dependence on CSSA as a result of having secured paid employment (Legco Panel on Welfare Services, 2005a).

An in-depth look at the program participants can be gleaned from a recent study conducted by the Chinese University of Hong Kong (CUHK). This study, commissioned by the Social Welfare Department (the author was involved as principal investigator), surveyed 1,782 low-income people and interviewed 65 people through in-depth interviews, focus groups, and visits to IEAPs (Tang et al., 2005). The CUHK study has concentrated on criteria that give more information about the quality of employment and self-reliance. That is, the criteria referred to low-income people's will to work and self-reliance, which play a part in sustaining enduring employment. In other words, this study aimed to tap IEAP participants' attitudes and values toward work and welfare.

The average age of the survey respondents was 42.3 years (Tang et al., 2005). About half (49.1%) of the respondents were female. Again, about half (50.6%) of them were born in Mainland China. On average, the respondents had lived in Hong Kong for 22.9 years. They were all able-bodied people, according to official definitions. A larger proportion (49.8%) of the respondents were married. Those parents, on average, had children between 10 and 14 years of age. And again, the great majority of the respondents had permanent residences (95.3%). The great majority (92.9%) of the respondents had employment experience. They had, on average, an employment experience of 175.8 months. They were most likely to have worked in catering occupations (20.0%). In the previous three years, they had, on average, worked 4.2 jobs, earned a monthly income of HK$5,128 (US $657) and worked 39.0 hours per week. The majority of the respondents had experience with themselves or their families receiving CSSA (90.0%). The average duration of receiving CSSA in the family was 3.2 years.

Satisfaction with the IEAP was moderately high among the respondents. The detailed distribution of IEAP participants with different levels of satisfaction with the IEAP showed that whereas more IEAP participants were rather satisfied, roughly equal numbers of ex-IEAP participants were rather satisfied and very satisfied (Table 4). Getting employment information (75.6%), receiving employment counseling (68.7%), and receiving job-matching (62.4%) were the most common services used by IEAP participants. In contrast, child-care services (2.1%) and home-care services (4.4%) were the least used. Getting a job

TABLE 4. Percentages of Satisfaction with the IEAP in Hong Kong

	IEAP (n = 473)					Ex-IEAP (n = 118)				
	Very dissatisfied	Dissatisfied	Neutral	Rather satisfied	Very satisfied	Very dissatisfied	Dissatisfied	Neutral	Rather satisfied	Very satisfied
Satisfaction	3.7	7.9	35.3	37.5	15.6	0.0	4.3	27.2	44.6	23.9

Source: Tang et al. (2005), page 50.

after joining the IEAP was significantly more likely among ex-participants (64.6%) than among ongoing participants at the time of the survey (30.7%).

Some major findings could be noted. Firstly, comparing the current IEAP participants with ex-IEAP participants, their employment rate was 90% for the ex-IEAP participant and 23% for the current IEAP participants. The cumulative duration of employment for the ex-IEAP participants was 3.4 months and the hours working in the job per week were 47 hours. Their monthly earnings were HK$5,669 (US $726). Average IEAP participants and ex-IEAP participants, compared with non-participants or other CSSA recipients, were more likely to have the following characteristics or beliefs: less inclined to depend on CSSA in the future; more supportive of self-reliance, more in favor of promoting work motivation, more motivated to find a job, more wanting to promote the importance of human and social capital, more likely to believe that they had job skills, more knowledgeable and confident about finding employment, and more believing that they had received assistance from others. Some success factors of the program were identified: IEAP participants who received temporary financial assistance (i.e., travel grants for job interviews, etc.) were more supportive of self-reliance and they regarded traveling expenses as less of an obstacle to employment. Besides, certain services provided by NGOs such as counseling related/not directly related to employment, job-seeking skill training and other training not directly related to employment, as well as post-employment support had positive impacts on participants' motivation and commitment to work.

Finally, the study finds that the more help and satisfaction a participant derived from the IEAP, the more the participant's commitment to self-reliance and work improved. It has to be noted that not every aspect of the IEAP is successful. Receiving job training, job-matching, job attachment and child-care and home-care services in the IEAPs did not generally show a favorable effect on the participant's welfare and work attitudes. It is fair to conclude that the IEAPs have made some differences in the lives of the able-bodied unemployed CSSA recipients.

Other than the survey, this study conducted a number of personal interviews of IEAP participants, CSSA single parents, ex-CSSA persons, and employers, as well as focus group discussions with government's Community Work practitioners, government's practitioners not involved in the Community Work, and the public. There were a total of 68 interviewees. Some good practices were identified for the IEAP: job variety, job placement, and networking with employers. Social workers' commitment of the NGOs was the most common merit identified for IEAPs. Accordingly, staff commitment could lead to a demonstrative effect on participants, who might raise their work motivation.

Understandably, the study showed that there was a preference for NGOs to operate IEAPs among the social welfare practitioners. Some reasons were cited for this preference: NGOs' comprehensive and territory- or region-wide services in support of employment; the independence of employment assistance from providing CSSA and imposing sanctions on receiving it; and having no need to identify participants as CSSA recipients. The latter reason helped participants find jobs when they would not suffer from stigmatization associated with receiving CSSA (Tang et al., 2005).

CONCLUDING REMARKS

The East Asian crisis led to serious poverty and prompted their governments to reconsider the status of their welfare program. Ideally, the primary goal of poverty/inequality reduction efforts would be to increase the well-being of East Asian people living in poverty–through projects, programs, policy level interventions and institution building that will systematically reduce poverty and eliminate the root causes of poverty. All of these efforts can lead to poverty reduction if governments can identify and articulate the root causes of poverty, make the links between what they are doing to ameliorate the situation and who will benefit, understand how and why poor people make decisions and ensure that stakeholders are involved in local planning processes (Tang & Wong, 2003). As noted earlier, Asian states preferred to rely on renewed economic growth and some temporary measures to tackle the social need problem. In the case of Hong Kong, this approach was augmented by the introduction of a series of welfare to work programs since 1998.

Eight years after the Asian crisis, Hong Kong is still facing its adverse repercussions. Its welfare system is still under strain. For instance, CSSA unemployment cases have increased over nine times from 4,866 at the end of 1994 to 45,231 at the end of 2004, while the number of low earnings cases have increased 17 times from 947 to 16,176 during the same period. Thus, in terms of sheer number, 93,956 CSSA recipients are in the unemployment category and 63,842 are in the low earnings category as of May 2005 (Legco Panel on Welfare Services, 2005a). The pressure is now on the SAR government to look for effective ways to tackle the problem of unemployment and the rising number of people on welfare.

This paper argues that the IEAPs, one of the core welfare to work programs, have been somewhat effective in enabling CSSA recipients to return to the market. According to the Social Welfare Department's statistics, Batch 1 of the IEAPs (40 of the 105 projects) assisted 46.2% of the participants in securing full-time employment, 13.1% of the CSSA recipients in leaving the CSSA net, 23.8% in changing to low-earnings status, and 28.9% in securing employment over three months.

Inevitably, one could conclude from these findings that early and intensive intervention in the form of employment and personal assistance from professional social workers has induced positive value and attitudinal changes (e.g., job motivation and a willingness to find a job) on the recipients' part. Practically, these findings echo those done in many advanced industrialized countries like the United States and Britain on welfare to work programs (Bryson, 2003; Blundell, 2001, cited in Bryson).

Despite these findings, there are several cautionary notes. As argued by many academics, economic effects of the welfare to work programs in the advanced nations like the United States have been encouraging, but these programs are implemented in the context of a rapidly growing economy (Bryson, 2003; Lehrer et al., 2002; Midgley & Tang, 2001). Therefore the cause of the reduction was most likely the economic boom rather than the success of workfare. According to recent U.S. experiences, there is little evidence to support the belief that welfare reform based on a "work-first" model *alone* can magically solve the problems of poverty and deprivation (Midgley, 1999). The work-first approach of workfare, especially in providing no training or counseling to welfare recipients, is particularly problematic and unlikely to be effective (Midgley & Tang, 2001). The desired approach tends to be one committed to developing recipients' employability and human capital. This approach would be consistent with the IEAP, which offers job training and counseling. Hence, the IEAP can take credit for promoting self-reliance and employment through development of human capital.

On the other hand, tough critics of welfare to work program in North America (Snyder, 2003; Abramovitz, 1997) question the overall values of welfare to work programs. Thus Abramovitz (1997) alludes to a dilemma in the welfare to work program:

> Some non-profit agencies provide useful training experiences for one or more workfare participants, but cooperating with workfare programs may bring harm to the large majority of recipients. Can the non-profits train all the 10,000 workfare participants in the non-profit pipeline? What about those among the thousands of recipients who are in less protected settings in non-profit or city agencies? Do the benefits for a few outweigh the human costs of a program that keeps the poor from large-scale education and training programs that might actually lift them out of poverty and off welfare?

These comments merit serious debate that goes beyond the purview of this paper. However, it is a pity that many critics seldom articulate clear and sustainable policy alternatives to existing welfare to work programs, other than putting a renewed emphasis on increasing social transfers, a condition that is difficult to attain given dwindling public resources. While the IEAPs in Hong Kong have some positive results, one must admit that a "work-first" model is not a cure-all. Policies that promote sustained economic growth and the capability for full participation in the economy would be necessary. A "social investment approach" aims at investing in individuals, families, and the community to enhance their capacity to cope with changes and adversities, to seek to maximize individuals' strengths, and to promote self-reliance and self-betterment. A key feature of this approach is strong reliance on resources from the government, the third sector and the business sector (i.e., tripartite partnership). This approach has become popular in contemporary policy debates (Midgley & Tang, 2001; Midgley & Sherraden, 2000; Midgley, 1999, 1997, 1995). In place of responding to the quests for rights and needs, the social investment approach aspires to develop people's capabilities and thus enable people to participate in the economy actively.

This approach urges governments to assume responsibility for directing economic growth in ways that are sustainable and that promote social well-being for all. It also calls on governments to emphasize social programs that are compatible with development. Central to its conception of social progress through development, it stresses two key underlying principles: first, economic development should be integrated and sustainable, bringing benefits to all citizens; and second, social welfare should be investment-oriented (i.e., "productivist welfare"), seeking to enhance human capacities to participate in the economy (Midgley, 1995, 1999).

The productivist welfare approach in social development emphasized the adoption of social policies that strive to enhance human functioning and capabilities. Central programmatic provisions include investments in human capital, employment and self-employment programs, social capital formation, asset development, and the removal of barriers to economic participation (Midgley, 1995, 1997). In this respect, employment and other activities are keys to sustaining people's dignity and well-being and safeguarding equality in society. Accordingly, the crux of equality rests on the economic participation of all people, rather than having equal shares of resources. This broader framework would be better able to address the needs of the welfare clients and the members of deprived, low-income communities in Hong Kong.

There is an added significance to this approach. The productivist welfare approach promotes a consensual model (Tang & Midgley, 2002; Midgley, 1995). The major stakeholders involved in promoting social development include the state, the community, non-governmental organizations, employers and workers. The involvement of these different groups is very important to the post-colonial Hong Kong that has been threatened by lingering unemployment and inequities and where social and political divisions are becoming more marked (Tang & Wong, 2003; Tang & Midgley, 2002). By involving many constituencies in both economic and social policy, the prospects of reviving social solidarity and promoting social integration increase.

REFERENCES

Abramovitz, M. (1997). *Workfare and the non-profits? Myths and realities.* Task Force on Welfare Reform, NYC Chapter, NASW. Retrieved on November 18, 2005 from *http://www.sullivan-county.com/id2/workfare_myth.htm.*

Blundell, R. (2001a). Welfare to work: Which policies work and why? *Keynes Lecture in Economics.* London: University College London and Institute for Fiscal Studies.

Blundell, R. (2001b). Welfare reform for low income workers. *Oxford Economics Papers, 53,* 18-214.

Bryson, A. (2003). From welfare to workfare. In Jane Millar (Ed.), *Understanding social security* (pp. 77-102). Bristol: The Policy Press.

Chow, N. W. S. (2003). New economy and new social policy in East and Southeast Asian compact, mature economies: The case of Hong Kong. *Social Policy and Administration, 37*(4): 411-422.

Commission of Poverty (2005). *Comprehensive social security assistance scheme: Able-bodied caseload–Past trend and 2014 scenarios.* Hong Kong: The Author.

Cooney, S. (1999). Testing times for the ILO: Institutional reform for the new international political economy. *Comparative Labor Law and Policy Journal, 20*(3): 365-400.

Council of Economic Advisers (1999). *The effects of welfare policy and the economic expansion on welfare caseloads: An update.* Washington, DC. Retrieved on November 18, 2005 from: *http://ftp.fedworld.gov/pub/w-house/0814-6.txt*

Dahl, E. (2003). Does workfare work? The Norwegian Experience. *International Journal of Social Welfare, 12,* 274-288.

Fraser, A., & Nyland, C. (1997). In search of the middle way: The ILO, standard setting and globalization. *Australian Journal of Labour Law, 10,* 280-286.

Goodman, R., White, G., & Kwon, H. (1998). *The East Asian welfare model: Welfare Orientalism and the state.* New York: Routledge.

Holtz, T. H. (1999). Labour rights are human rights. *Lancet, 353*(9156), 923.

International Labor Organization (ILO) (1999). *Social issues arising from the East Asia economic crisis and policy implications for the future.* Discussion summary prepared by Katherine Hagen, ILO Deputy Director-General, January 21-22, Bangkok ILO Regional Meeting. Retrieved on November 18, 2005 from *http://www.worldbank.org/eapsocial/meeting/ilo.htm*

International Monetary Fund (IMF) (1999). *The IMF's response to the Asian crisis. A fact sheet, January 17.* Retrieved on November 18, 2005 from *http://imf.org/External/np/exr/facts/asia.HTM.*

International Social Service Hong Kong Branch (ISSHKB) (2005). *Intensive employment assistance projects.* Retrieved on November 18, 2005, from *http://www.isshk.org/Annual%20Report%202004/ train.html*

Legislative Council (Legco) Panel on Welfare Services, Subcommittee on Review of the Comprehensive Social Security Assistance Scheme (2005a). *Evaluation study of the Intensive Employment Assistance Projects for Comprehensive Social Security Assistance (CSSA) and near-CSSA recipients.* Hong Kong: Hong Kong SAR Government.

Legislative Council (Legco) Panel on Welfare Services, Subcommittee on Review of the Comprehensive Social Security Assistance Scheme (2005b). *The review of arrangements for single parent recipients under the Comprehensive Social Security Assistance Scheme.* Hong Kong: Hong Kong SAR Government.

Lehrer, E., Crittenden, K., & Norr, K. F. (2002). Depression and economic self-sufficiency among inner-city minority mothers. *Social Science Research, 31,* 285-301.

Leung, K., Ip, O., & Au, K. (2003). *Evaluation of the Ending Exclusion Project for Social Welfare Department.* Hong Kong: Social Welfare Department.

Midgley, J. (1986). Industrialization and welfare: The case of the four little tigers. *Social Policy and Administration. 20,(4):* 225-238.

Midgley, J. (1995). *Social development: The developmental perspective in social welfare*. Thousand Oaks, CA: Sage.

Midgley, J. (1997). *Social welfare in global context*. Thousand Oaks, CA: Sage.

Midgley, J. (1999). Growth, redistribution and welfare: Towards social investment. *Social Service Review, 77*(1), 3-2.

Midgley, J., & Sherraden, M. (2000). The social development perspective in social policy. In J. Midgley, M. B. Tracy, & M. Livermore (Eds.), *The handbook of social policy* (pp. 435-446). Thousand Oaks, CA: Sage Publications.

Midgley, J., & Tang, K. L. (2001). Introduction: Social policy, economic growth and developmental welfare. *International Journal of Social Welfare. 10*(4), 244-252.

Morgen, S., & Maskovsky, J. (2003). The anthropology of welfare reform: New perspectives on U.S. poverty in the post-welfare era. *Annual Review of Anthropology, 32,* 315-338.

Noel, A. (1995). The politics of workfare. In Adil Sayeed (Ed.), *Workfare: Does It work? Is it fair?* (pp. 39-73). Montreal, Canada: Institute for Research on Public Policy.

Organization of Economic Cooperation and Development (OECD) (2000). *Pushing ahead with reform in Korea: Labour market and social safety net policies*. Paris: OECD.

Peck, J. (2002). Political economics of scale: Fast policy, inter-scalar relations, and neoliberal workfare. *Economic Geography, 78*(3), 331-360.

Snyder, L. (2003). Workfare. In A. Westhues (Ed.) *Canadian social policy: Issues and perspectives* (pp. 108-127). Toronto: Wilfrid Laurier University Press.

Social Welfare Department, Hong Kong (2001). *"Support for self-reliance" Scheme for comprehensive social security assistance for unemployed recipients* (Final Evaluation Report). Hong Kong: Author.

Social Welfare Department, Hong Kong (2005). *Support for self-reliance.* Retrieved on November 21, 2005 from *http://www.info.gov.hk/swd/html _eng/whatsnew/doc/ 08_03/230703.ppt*

Tang, K. L. (1998). *Colonial state and social policy: Social welfare development in Hong Kong 1842-1997*. Lanham, MD: University of America Press.

Tang, K. L. (2000a). *Social welfare development in East Asia*. New York: St. Martin's Press.

Tang, K.L. (2000b). Asian crisis, social welfare, and policy responses: Hong Kong and Korea compared. *International Journal of Sociology and Social Policy, 20*(5-6): 49-71.

Tang, K. L., & Midgley, J. (2002). Social policy after the East Asian crisis: Forging a normative basis for welfare. *Journal of Asian Comparative Development, 1*(2): 301-318.

Tang, K. L., & Wong, C. K. (Eds.) (2003). *Poverty monitoring and alleviation in East Asia*. New York: Nova Science Press.

Tang, K. L., Mok, B. H., Cheung, J. C. K., & Lou, V. W. Q. (2005). *An evaluation study of intensive employment assistance projects for CSSA and near-CSSA recipients* (Draft Report). Hong Kong: Department of Social Welfare.

Wilding, P. (1996). *Social policy and social development in Hong Kong*. Working Paper Series 1996/3, City University of Hong Kong, Department of Applied Social Studies.

The Role of Social Workers
in Welfare to Work Programs:
International Perspectives
on Policy and Practice

Jane Millar
Michael J. Austin

SUMMARY. Welfare to work is an important arena for understanding the changing nature of social policy and practice in Australia, the UK, Hong Kong, and the United States. This article discusses some key policy and practice issues in respect to social work professional training and practice. Welfare to work programs focus on "active" measures and stress the importance of "responsibilities" for all people of working age to support themselves through employment. The programs are being implemented in different ways across these different countries but in all cases the focus is increasingly on groups of people who may require sub-

Jane Millar, PhD, is Professor of Social Policy, Department of Social and Policy Sciences, University of Bath, Claverton Down, BATH BA2 7AY United Kingdom (E-mail: hssjim@bath.ac.uk).

Michael J. Austin, PhD, is Professor of Management and Planning, School of Social Welfare, University of California, Berkeley, 120 Haviland Hall, Berkeley, CA 94704 (E-mail: mjaustin@berkeley.edu).

[Haworth co-indexing entry note]: "The Role of Social Workers in Welfare to Work Programs: International Perspectives on Policy and Practice." Millar, Jane, and Michael J. Austin. Co-published simultaneously in *Journal of Policy Practice* (The Haworth Press, Inc.) Vol. 5, No. 2/3, 2006, pp. 149-158; and: *International Perspectives on Welfare to Work Policy* (ed: Richard Hoefer, and James Midgley) The Haworth Press, Inc., 2006, pp. 149-158. Single or multiple copies of this article are available for a fee from The Haworth Document Delivery Service [1-800-HAWORTH, 9:00 a.m. - 5:00 p.m. (EST). E-mail address: docdelivery@ haworthpress.com].

Available online at http://www.haworthpress.com/web/JPP
doi:10.1300/J508v05n02_10

stantial levels of assistance to meet their needs and to help them find and sustain employment. *[Article copies available for a fee from The Haworth Document Delivery Service: 1-800-HAWORTH. E-mail address: <docdelivery@ haworthpress.com> Website: <http://www.HaworthPress.com> © 2006 by The Haworth Press, Inc. All rights reserved.]*

KEYWORDS. Welfare to work, comparative social policy, Australia, UK, Hong Kong, US

INTRODUCTION

As the articles in this special volume have shown, welfare to work is an important arena for understanding the changing nature of social policy and practice in Australia, the UK, Hong Kong, and the United States. The symposium ended with a round-table discussion of the issues arising from these national case studies. In this final article we reflect on some of the cross-cutting themes that have emerged out of the presentation of these "progress reports" on welfare to work programs in these four countries. One of the aims of the symposium was to explore the role of professionally educated social workers in the welfare to work programs in these countries. In general, it was found that this role is limited. However, our discussions highlighted two main areas where a social work agenda could, and should, be further developed: (1) the identification of public policy themes that would benefit from increased social work involvement with respect to policy development, and (2) the role of practice in policy implementation.

PUBLIC POLICY THEMES

"Welfare to work" is a shorthand term used for a range of policies aimed at getting non-employed people into paid work. While this has always been one of the objectives of social and economic policy, the current focus on paid work as the most important and central policy goal appears to represent a paradigmatic change in the nature of the social welfare systems in these as well as other countries. The policy shifts include: (1) from promoting "rights" to benefits to "responsibilities" associated with benefits, (2) from "passive" social policy based on eligibility to "active" social policies based on "work first," and (3) from the "social protection" of individuals and families with dependent children to the "social inclusion" of all eligible citizens. These shifts represent profound changes in the nature, meaning and activities of the welfare state in the 21st century.

However, there are also significant cross-national differences in what welfare to work means in practice. At least three key differences can be noted for these countries. First, there are differences in the way that the target groups are defined. In the USA, it is single mothers (lone parents) who are the key target group. In the other countries, the focus is more on long-term unemployed people or on unemployed youth, and lone mothers are usually included in welfare to work policies but are not the most important target group. Secondly, there are differences in the extent to which compulsion is embedded in these policies. Again, the USA is different, with a mandatory system in which work has indeed *replaced* welfare for most potential recipients, such that some engagement with work is a condition of welfare receipt and sanctions are applied to those who do not comply. In the other countries the extent of compulsion varies for different groups of people; generally, the highest degree of compulsion is applied to those who are unemployed, especially the long-term unemployed, and other groups–such as disabled people, lone mothers, etc.–are usually included on a voluntary basis. Thirdly, there are significant differences in the "welfare mix" in terms of public, private and voluntary sector involvement in both the funding and delivery of these services. For example, in Hong Kong the private sector has provided funding for pilot programs, while in Australia the delivery of the labor market assistance is entirely contracted out to the private and voluntary sectors.

These differences reflect the importance of path dependency in structuring the ways in which reforms are developed and implemented. Path dependency in the development of social policies refers not only to the goals and aspirations of policymakers but also to the previous history of social policy, the nature of institutional structures used to implement social policy, and the cultural and political values of the larger society. In essence, national identities shape policy options and choices and even radical reform is a *reform* of what is already in existence. As a result, welfare provisions reflect the values of the society in which they are developed and cross-national comparisons demonstrate how social policies are defined differently in different countries.

On the other hand, our small world is in many ways getting smaller and these case studies also reflect the importance of policy transfer whereby ideas are transplanted from one country to another. This is true with respect to the ideological basis of these policies as well as the specific provisions being introduced. Research and evaluation have also been an important influence, especially for government policy leaders eager to learn from the experiences of others. However, the lessons learned by others are fraught with dangers when seeking local or country-specific application; for example, the evidence may be less than robust, the wrong conclusions may be drawn, and the importance of context underestimated.

One of the main aims of the symposium was to explore the different approaches to the implementation of welfare to work programs, especially the role of social workers in program administration and "case management" or "casework" support services. Again, there were substantial differences across the countries. In Australia social workers have been involved in the delivery of income maintenance programs for some years, taking an advocacy role, working in community development and working with staff to improve delivery. The welfare to work programs have led to some redefinition of the social worker role that has emerged out of the tension between the traditional social work values of promoting personal development and autonomy for program participants and the "work-first" goals of achieving employment target outcomes and utilizing sanctions for non-compliance. In Hong Kong social workers have become increasingly involved in welfare to work programs, partly as an opportunity to engage in welfare reform debates and poverty-related work. In the USA and the UK, by contrast, there is very little direct involvement by university-educated social workers in these programs, and services are often provided by career civil servants with little or no social work education.

In making links to the wider policy context, it is clear that labor market and wage policies are very important. In the US, in particular, there is very little recognition of links between child welfare, poverty and income support systems. The UK, however, is implementing welfare to work in the context of a specific national anti-poverty policy goal that is expressed in terms of the elimination of *child* poverty. This means that the British emphasis, although also oriented to the "work- first" model, includes a greater focus on issues of income and well-being in work than in the US. In essence, welfare to work programs in the US have lost their focus on protecting dependent children (the old AFDC, Aid to Families with Dependent Children was replaced in 1996 with TANF, Temporary Assistance to Needy Families) and the child welfare system has not yet incorporated the goal of family self-sufficiency as a key element in child protection.

And finally, it is important to assess the extent to which welfare to work policy developments are in tune with public opinion. In general, there does seem to be public support for the "rights/responsibilities" approach to income support programs where society values paid employment and devalues and/or stigmatizes those without work. Many people without paid work want to work and often welcome the help that they can receive under these programs. However, the extent of public support for employment obligations and the compulsion to enforce them varies across countries and among different groups of people in need (youth vs. lone mothers). In particular, there are very different views about the right balance between child rearing (care work inside the home) and paid work outside the home, especially in relationship to lone mothers. Obligations for single mothers to work full time, as in the USA, are likely to place immense pressure on their capacity to also provide care for their children, even if public child care was substantially expanded.

However, there may be strong public support for other ways of defining "responsibilities," beyond the paid work model. The concept of an "ethics of care," for example, is based on valuing the interdependence of people and on the need to structure social policy to take account of the interrelationship between care-giving and care-receiving over the life course (Sevenhuijsen, 1998). The concept of "social investment" is also based on recognition of the importance of interdependence among and between individuals, generations and society (Esping-Andersen, Gallie, Hemerijck, & Myers, 2002). In these approaches, welfare rights are viewed as collective rights for the benefit of society as a whole and not simply as individual entitlements. Social policy is never simply a technical exercise in "what works"; it is always about political choices and ideological values.

PRACTICE PERSPECTIVES

It is well-known that the professional backgrounds of persons in senior policy positions in government can have a significant impact on the multiple administrative guidelines generated to implement public policy. For example, during the 1960s and 1970s in the US, social workers held senior positions in the federal Children's Bureau and greatly influenced the direction of service delivery and the educational funding for preparing future practitioners. A similar pattern can now be seen in Australia with respect to implementing welfare to work programs that are guided by senior social workers in the national government. However, today it appears that the reforms in national welfare to work programs in the US and UK are being implemented by senior policy officials with backgrounds in economics and political science and little experience in delivering services to poor people. Until more social workers are educated and advance their careers into senior positions in welfare to work programs, this situation is not likely to change. So, how might social workers be better prepared to assume leadership roles related to the critical issues of poverty reduction and work enhancement? Two practice domains seem relevant to this analysis: (1) policy practice, and (2) service delivery.

Policy Practice

Examples of policy practice can be found in the numerous policy papers generated in the UK to refine and improve the implementation of the New Deal for Lone Parents program, such as giving personal advisors more discretion in the implementation of the voluntary welfare to work program for single mothers. This approach to policy practice suggests that ongoing policy analysis is a form of continuous value clarification in the UK, often expressed in the form of government policy papers that provide administrative guidelines. This unusual form of review and clarification is based on a demonstrated commitment to monitor the policy implementation process that reflects the evolving values of the welfare state.

In addition to this top-down perspective of policy practice, there is also a bottom-up view that seeks to minimize discrimination and stigmatization by collecting data from service users, especially efforts to understand the life-cycle of service users and adjust the implementation of public policy accordingly. For example, the implementation of welfare to work programs in Hong Kong reflects a tri-focal perspective that includes the client, the community, and government policymakers. The goals include advocating for the needs of client populations through community advocacy organizations that seek to influence the development and implementation of public policy. When it became clear that there were limits to the effectiveness of welfare to work programs (e.g., caseload reduction), efforts were made to establish a Poverty Alleviation Commission to address the root causes that led to the need for welfare programs.

Policy practice also involves worker discretion in the implementation of public policy, frequently referred to as the role of "street-level bureaucrats" (Lipsky, 1980). The issue of discretion is played out in multiple ways. At the front-line level, it involves efforts on the part of staff employed in welfare to work programs to either find multiple ways to be of assistance to those in need (the social work perspective) or to find ways to limit benefits (the taxpayer accountability perspective demonstrated by government bureaucrats). Discretion is also found at the managerial level where efforts are made either to contract with local service providers who have expertise relevant to the client population or to use contracting to reduce costs and devolve policy implementation authority from the national (or state) government to community-based non-profit organizations (Austin, 2003). The use of discretion in implementing public policy at the worker levels or at the managerial levels represents another way in which values permeate the implementation of welfare to work programs.

Aside from involving the business community in promoting a "work first" public policy approach to help the unemployed enter the workforce, the domain of policy practice can also include engaging the private sector in funding special programs. As demonstrated in the case of Hong Kong, funding from the Jockey Clubs represents the unusual entry of private philanthropy into the domain of welfare to work program design and innovation.

Service Delivery

Issues of service delivery are rooted in both an understanding of the role of work in the lives of different client populations and the role of education in the lives of social work students. As noted in both of the articles in this book on clients with learning difficulties and those with mental illness, paid work can be a central part of service delivery and the promotion of self-worth. Similarly, the crossover services in child welfare reflect the tensions of helping mothers who are having difficulty parenting their children while also trying to maintain employment. The role of work or employment in the lives of different client populations may not receive sufficient attention by service providers. Similarly, the collective voices of service users (advocacy organizations) provide additional challenges for service providers who are accustomed to dealing with clients as part of a caseload rather than as a population of citizens with rights and responsibilities.

Some of the most profound challenges emerging out of welfare to work programs relate to the education of future social workers. While there are significant differences in the ways in which social work students are educated in the countries represented by the articles in this volume, the common denominator appears to be related to the two concepts of "poverty" and "work." While an understanding of poverty has been an important foundation for the education of social workers over the past century, it is not clear how this theme appears in current university social work curricula and how extensively it is treated. While it is difficult to imagine social policy courses that do not mention poverty, to what extent does it receive attention beyond income maintenance policies and programs? While the social science knowledge base that contributes to our understanding of poverty is extensive (anthropology, sociology, economics, psychology, and political science), to what extent are social work students exposed to the breadth and depth of this issue? Similarly, while research on low-income employment, labor markets, and wage policy has relevance for those receiving social services, how extensively are these topics treated in a traditional social work program of study?

Other areas of relevant curriculum content relate to the teaching of human behavior and the social environment (HB&SE), research, and fieldwork. While the relevance of the social and behavioral sciences for social work practice is considerable, it is not clear that HB&SE courses include theories relevant to welfare to work programs. For example, a discussion of client help-seeking behaviors can be expanded to explore the research on job-seeking behaviors. Similarly, both client identity formation and worker identity formation are involved in the process of assisting unemployed people find and sustain work. Both clients and workers are shaped by their experiences with employment. In addition, the organizational factors involved in implementing welfare to work programs are significant for both the client and the workers. For example, when does coercion operate under the guise of empathy? How are decision-making styles affected (e.g., enforcers or enablers, trust-seekers or trust-builders, worthiness testers or empowerment promoters, social history seekers or champions of future possibilities)? As noted earlier, worker adaptations are captured in the research on "street-level bureaucrats" and are also referred to as "managerialism" in the British and Australian context when it comes to understanding the impact of business concepts on public sector programs. And finally, the multiple theories from different disciplines about the nature of work in our societies are central to a social work student's understanding of human behavior and the social environment.

Beyond human behavior and the social environment, all social work students are exposed to the importance of research methods. In some programs, students are expected to conduct an independent piece of research. It would be interesting to find out how much of this research each year addresses issues related to welfare to work programs. It is suspected that very few students pursue this area of research. Similarly, when it comes to selecting fieldwork learning opportunities, it is estimated that very few of them select welfare to work programs. In the UK this might be explained by the fact that local authority social service agencies have no responsibility for the national welfare to work programs, therefore providing little incentive for students placed in public or voluntary sector organizations to learn about welfare to work programs. In contrast, in the US the welfare to work programs can be found in either local county social service agencies or in state agencies related to social services or employment and training. In Australia, the learning opportunities in local welfare to work programs include a mixture of customer service delivery and community development (enhancing service networks through inter-agency coordination, partnership development, and micro-enterprise development in rural areas).

IMPLICATIONS AND CONCLUSIONS

These four national case studies of welfare to work policies and programs provided an opportunity to explore welfare reform at a number of different levels: rhetoric and discourse, policy goals and objectives, institutional structures and change, and service delivery and practice. This format provided a very rich agenda for analysis and discussion.

It is clear that policymakers in these countries have turned away from "passive" programs of cash support in order to promote welfare to work for as wide a spectrum of people as possible. This has meant an increasing focus on those who require greater levels of assistance to help them find and sustain employment. This is where the boundaries with social services become more apparent, but also more difficult. Those delivering these services are expected to focus on labor market outcomes, in particular job placements, but the people they are dealing with may need a much wider range of specialist support to help them find, and sustain, employment. As job brokers, welfare to work staff seek to reach target numbers for people placed in entry-level work, and their training and institutional support are unlikely to equip them for these wider or more specialist roles. On the other hand, social workers deal with poor people on a daily basis but their training and professional development appears not to provide an in-depth understanding of poverty and unemployment issues, and the obligations and requirements of public assistance. There is a considerable research, practice and training agenda to be developed in these areas, both for those who are developing policy and those who are delivering welfare to work services as well as those providing general social services. For example, a future research agenda might address the following policy and practice implications and questions:

Policy Implications. To what extent are welfare to work programs pro-family or anti-family in their implementation? To what extent has the goal of caseload reduction been a substitute for addressing poverty reduction?

Practice Implications. To what extent is a comprehensive understanding of poverty guiding the practice of those in welfare to work programs, and how many of the practitioners are trained social workers? To what extent do welfare to work programs call for community work strategies more than traditional casework strategies?

It is clear that the contributions in this volume raise important questions for the future.

REFERENCES

Austin, M.J. (2003). The changing relationship between non-profit organizations and public social service agencies in the era of welfare reform. *Nonprofit and Voluntary Sector Quarterly, 32*(1), 97-114.

Esping-Andersen, G., Gallie, D., Hemerijck, A., & Myers, J. (2002). *Why We Need a New Welfare State.* Oxford: Oxford University Press.

Lipsky, M. (1980). *Street-Level Bureaucracy: Dilemmas of the Individual in Public Services.* New York: Russell Sage Foundation.

Sevenhuijsen, S. (1998). *Citizenship and the Ethics of Care: Feminist Considerations on Justice, Morality and Politics.* London: Routledge.

Index

BOOK ORDER FORM!

Order a copy of this book with this form or online at:
http://www.HaworthPress.com/store/product.asp?sku= 5876

International Perspectives on Welfare to Work Policy

—— in softbound at $17.95 ISBN-13: 978-0-7890-3368-0 / ISBN-10: 0-7890-3368-2.
—— in hardbound at $37.95 ISBN-13: 978-0-7890-3367-3 / ISBN-10: 0-7890-3367-4.

COST OF BOOKS _____

POSTAGE & HANDLING _____
US: $4.00 for first book & $1.50
for each additional book
Outside US: $5.00 for first book
& $2.00 for each additional book.

SUBTOTAL _____

In Canada: add 7% GST. _____

STATE TAX _____
CA, IL, IN, MN, NJ, NY, OH, PA & SD residents
please add appropriate local sales tax

FINAL TOTAL _____
If paying in Canadian funds, convert
using the current exchange rate,
UNESCO coupons welcome.

❑ **BILL ME LATER:**
Bill-me option is good on US/Canada/
Mexico orders only; not good to jobbers,
wholesalers, or subscription agencies.

❑ **Signature** _____

❑ **Payment Enclosed: $**_____

❑ **PLEASE CHARGE TO MY CREDIT CARD:**
❑ Visa ❑ MasterCard ❑ AmEx ❑ Discover
❑ Diner's Club ❑ Eurocard ❑ JCB

Account #_____

Exp Date_____

Signature_____
(Prices in US dollars and subject to change without notice.)

PLEASE PRINT ALL INFORMATION OR ATTACH YOUR BUSINESS CARD

Name _____

Address _____

City _____ State/Province _____ Zip/Postal Code _____

Country _____

Tel _____ Fax _____

E-Mail _____

May we use your e-mail address for confirmations and other types of information? ❑Yes ❑No We appreciate receiving
your e-mail address. Haworth would like to e-mail special discount offers to you, as a preferred customer.
We will never share, rent, or exchange your e-mail address. We regard such actions as an invasion of your privacy.

Order from your **local bookstore** or directly from
The Haworth Press, Inc. 10 Alice Street, Binghamton, New York 13904-1580 • USA
Call our toll-free number (1-800-429-6784) / Outside US/Canada: (607) 722-5857
Fax: 1-800-895-0582 / Outside US/Canada: (607) 771-0012
E-mail your order to us: orders@HaworthPress.com

For orders outside US and Canada, you may wish to order through your local
sales representative, distributor, or bookseller.
For information, see http://HaworthPress.com/distributors

(Discounts are available for individual orders in US and Canada only, not booksellers/distributors.)

Please photocopy this form for your personal use.
www.HaworthPress.com

BOF06